I'm Lazy and I Love to Eat

I'm Lazy and I Love to Eat

Mary T. Prenon

ISBN-13: 9781548326746
ISBN-10: 1548326747
Library of Congress Control Number: 2017910156
CreateSpace Independent Publishing Platform
North Charleston, South Carolina

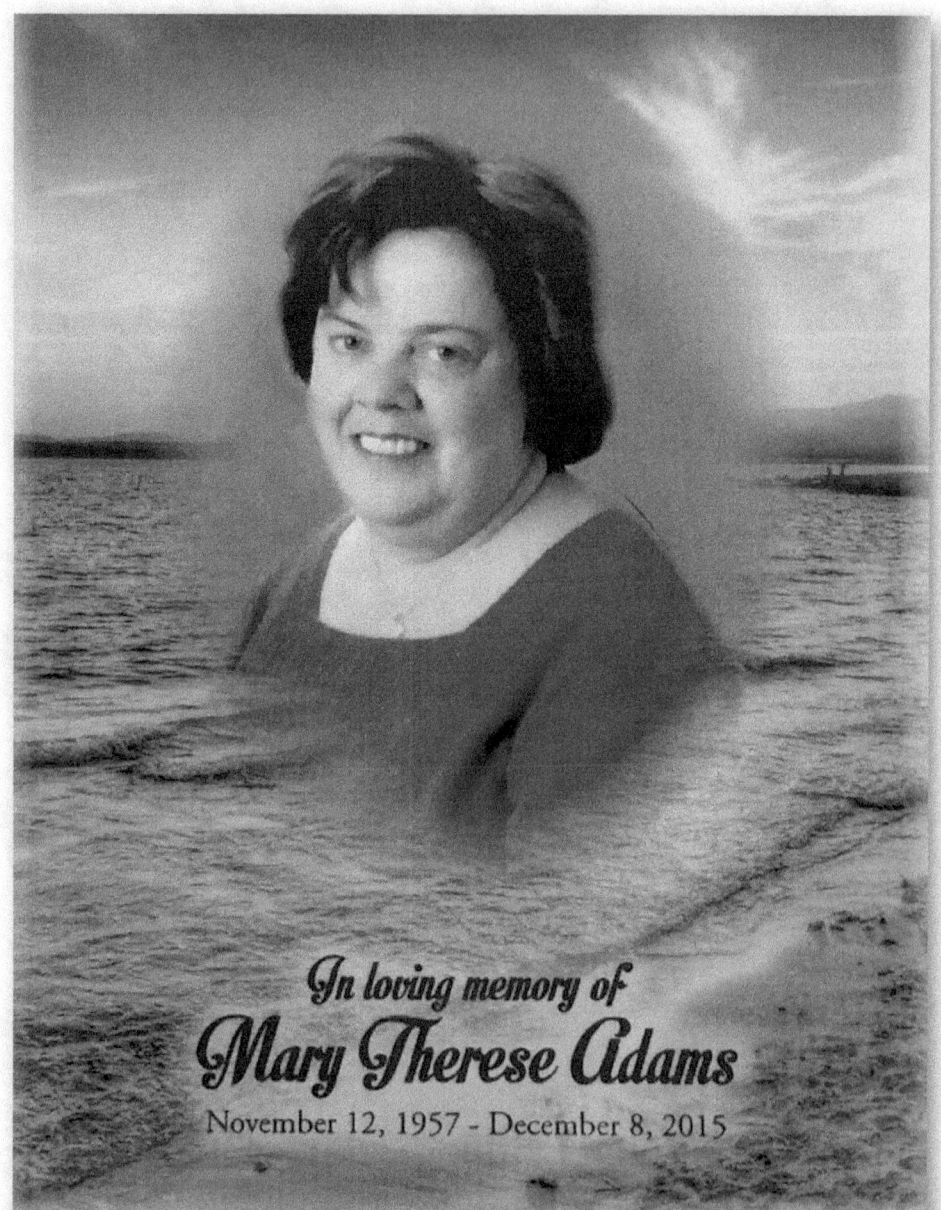

In loving memory of

Mary Therese Adams

November 12, 1957 - December 8, 2015

Dedication

This book is dedicated to my best friend, the late, great Mary Adams, or "Madam," as we liked to call her. Madam passed away in December 2015 in a tragic car accident in Pennsylvania. She was just fifty-eight years old and way too young to leave us all.

Madam and I had been friends since we were seven years old, and one thing that we always enjoyed talking and laughing about was eating, gaining weight, trying to lose weight, getting frustrated, and then finally saying, "Screw it all!"

She knew about this book, and I think she'd be so proud and happy that I finally finished it after nineteen years. You will hear more about her and our friendship throughout this book.

Suffice it to say, not a day goes by that I don't think of her. Whenever I see a piece of cheesecake, I look up to the heavens, knowing that she's there eating every kind of cheesecake ever made and not gaining an ounce.

Here's to you, Madam. I couldn't have written this without you.

Thank You

want to say a special thank-you to my friend Paula Garber for editing this book and for believing that I would one day finish it. Paula and I worked together at a local advertising agency and were also in a writing group many years ago. It was in this group where I first disclosed that I was writing the book. Paula is a fantastic editor who does work for some very large and well-known publishing firms in New York City. I'm so happy that she wanted to be a part of this.

I also want to give special thanks to my friend Kate Borman, another ad agency alumna, who designed the cover of this book. Kate is an award-winning graphic artist who started her own company in 2014. Her insights into my wacky personality are very well represented in the cover.

Preface

One of the big questions that continues to plague our planet is, "Why is weight loss such a huge problem?" Losing weight and getting fit seem so very simple when you think about it. All you have to do is make healthy eating choices and exercise. Simple, right? Then why is "weight loss" a multibillion dollar industry? I'll tell you why—because most people are like me. They start out with great intentions, but then life gets in the way. When they don't see results quickly enough, they start to feel bad about themselves, get frustrated, cry, and quit. Then they start up again with some new fad diet, and the whole thing repeats itself—including the crying.

How do you recover and move on? How do you gear yourself up to go through the setbacks and disappointments? Here's the three-word answer: never give up. Remember, you fail only when you give up, so if you keep hanging in there, you'll never fail.

You also have to learn to laugh at yourself. While I know firsthand that working to go from fat to fit can be frustrating and depressing, I try to find something that's funny or makes me happy in every situation. So you swallow a pizza and inhale the last piece of cheesecake at a party—now there's a lasting memory for you and your friends.

I have many fond memories of using humor to help me deal with things throughout my struggle to the land of fitness. Once I went to one of those haunted houses at Halloween, and when a costumed ghoul came at me with a plastic meat cleaver, I pointed to my left thigh and begged him to take a little off the side.

I especially have to thank my dear friends Mary (a.k.a. "Madam") and Helen for keeping me laughing with our outrageous "I'm fatter than you are" stories. We'd call each other and tell tales of how we were so fat that the restaurant we were going to would have to widen the doors for us to get in. Sometimes we'd discuss how

Philadelphia's Walt Whitman Bridge and New York's George Washington Bridge had to be reinforced once we crossed over it, or how airplanes were unable to take off once we boarded them.

But here's a nice revelation. When I volunteered with a group providing free work clothing for people in need, I discovered that most women are *not* in the single-digit sizes. We had very few calls for sizes below 10, but a tremendous need for sizes twelve, fourteen, sixteen, and eighteen. So what does that tell you about the average American woman? One day, a couple of women looking through a box of pantyhose asked me if there were any queen sizes. As I started to help them look, one of the women picked up a pair of pantyhose and started reading the label. "One size fits all. Yeah, right," she said. "I've heard *that* before!" We all got a good laugh.

After years of frustration, tears, and a lot of laughing at myself, currently, at age sixty, I'm finally down from about 210 pounds to a manageable 160 pounds. (I'm still working on myself, and if I ever get down from to 150 again, I'll alert the media!) At just about five feet eight inches tall, I'm not skinny by any stretch of the imagination. I do not have a washboard stomach, and my arms, thighs, and butt still jiggle a bit. But so what? A little jiggling is a good thing. The bottom line is that I feel great and look decent, and my blood pressure and cholesterol levels are finally under control. My cardiologist has even stopped bugging the crap out of me to lose weight. (You'll hear more about him later.) Best of all, I'm done crying.

My goal in writing this book is to help you accomplish your goals—no matter how long it may take. This book is not a diet book or an exercise book. I don't have a background in nutrition or psychology. This is a real person's view of the problems we all face and how we can overcome them.

Believe me—it hasn't been easy, but after throwing crap against the wall long enough, something had to stick. There are no magic potions, no pills, no juices, no shakes, no protein bars, or any other bogus miracle diets that will make you shed pounds and get fit overnight. After all this time, my epiphany about the secret of weight loss and fitness can be summed up in two words: hard work.

Nobody wants to hear that, and that's why the diet industry will continue to flourish. Hell, for nineteen years I didn't want to hear it. Hard work? Really? There *must* be another way. Well, guess what? There isn't.

I finally realized that I needed to stop whining, suck it up, eat more veggies and less sugar, and get my fat butt to the gym. Yes, it sucks in the beginning, but if you stick with it, I guarantee it will stop sucking when you start to look and feel good. (Again, it took me almost twenty years to realize this!)

With that said, of course, I still have bad days—bad weeks even. But now I get up every day and do my best to make healthy eating choices and get in some form of exercise—even if it's mall walking. And, most importantly, having a healthy lifestyle doesn't mean giving up the cheesecake entirely. Once a week, I allow myself to eat what I want without going overboard. After all, life is too short.

I hope you enjoy this book. I want you to laugh at me, and I want you to be able to laugh at yourself when things don't go the way you expect. Most of all, I want to share my experiences and help you on your journey to a healthier lifestyle.

If this book helps just one person, it will give me more pleasure than a truckload of Boston cream pies. (Well, maybe.)

CHAPTER 1

Help! I'm Fat, and I Can't Get Thin!

As the title of this book suggests, I am a lazy sloth, and I love to eat. When I started writing this book in 1998, I was forty-one-years old and a good fifty or more pounds overweight. By some standards, I was even considered obese. (God, I hate that word.) The highest weight I ever saw on my scale was 198, but I knew I'd surpassed that when I could no longer fit into my extra-large-sized clothes. My guess is that my top weight was somewhere around 205 to 210. For months I'd go without weighing myself because I was terrified of seeing a number that would send me into a depressive tailspin.

I hated that damn scale and cried almost every time I stepped on it. The only thing I hated more than the scale was my body. I'd look in the mirror and cry. I'd put on clothes and cry. Hell, I'd even cry when I started to lose a tiny bit of weight because, in my mind, it was never enough, and I'd never look good.

Sometimes, I'd lose up to ten pounds, but then I'd reward myself with fatty, sugary foods and end up gaining it back. I thought rewarding myself like this was OK, and my reasoning was that it worked when I was in my twenties. News flash! My body had long outgrown its twenties.

On any given day, I felt like a human sandwich board, the body double for the *Baby Huey* cartoon character, or the poster child for the current month's issue of *Good Eatin' Magazine*. My waist was as big as the equator. My thighs were wiggling "jelly fests" topped with cellulite. My arms were canned hams, and my rear end, the prize rump roast at the county fair. I made it a point to avoid construction sites, afraid that one of the workers would slap a "Wide Load" sign on my ass. I dreaded going to the beach for fear of being jabbed with a harpoon (like a whale, get it?). OK, so I'm exaggerating a bit, but you get the picture.

Summer was the absolute worst time for being overweight. The rest of the year, I could hide my flab under big sweaters and overcoats, but unfortunately, I couldn't wear a parka to the beach. Every spring I swore that I'd be fit by the summer, and every summer I would squeeze into elastic-waist shorts and find the most body-camouflaging beach cover-ups. I hated having my picture taken—especially in the summer. I would look at the photo and then swear that it wasn't me. I developed an automatic flight response any time I saw anyone with a camera.

I'd often use the excuse that it was genetics. Both of my parents were slightly overweight, but not obese. So how did I become so "nutritionally challenged" (a.k.a. fat)? When I was born, I was so small—4.8 pounds—that my parents had to leave me in the hospital for a week until I reached five pounds. I was born about a month premature, and Mom always said I was impatient from the day I emerged from the womb. (Hey, I had places to crawl and people to meet!)

My life began in suburban Philadelphia in 1957, when there were no diet sodas, low-fat cookies, or health clubs. The words "Internet" and "cell phone" were nonexistent at that time, and "social media" meant going outside to talk to your neighbors.

I attended the local Catholic elementary school and ate lots of sugary treats and soft pretzels at recess. The nuns would always ask for volunteers to sell the candy at recess, and of course, I loved to volunteer for that. (If I couldn't sell it all, I would just eat it and ask my parents for the money!)

I vacationed at the New Jersey shore, eating tons of cotton candy, ice cream, and pizza. Ironically, I never gained weight back then because there was the great outdoors and games like tag, toys like hula-hoops, and activities like roller-skating, ice-skating, and bike riding. No matter what I ate as a child, I remained quite thin.

In 1971, when I started high school at age fourteen, I was still skinny. Back then I don't think they made uniforms in plus sizes, so you either fit into the standard sizes, or you were out of luck.

On summer nights, the neighborhood kids would get together and play games like Jailer (a mix of Tag and Hide-and-Go-Seek), Charge, (basically running across a lawn and hoping not to be tagged), and Wire Ball (throwing a ball in the air to try to hit the telephone wires). Then we'd make our nightly trek down to the local deli where we could get a cream soda and chips for only fifty cents. Sometimes, when it was really hot, we'd sit around and listen to the radio or play records (no CDs or iPods, just vinyl).

Sometime between the ages of fourteen and fifteen, the nasty scourge of acne slowly moved in on my face. For the next several years, I was a dermatologist's dream,

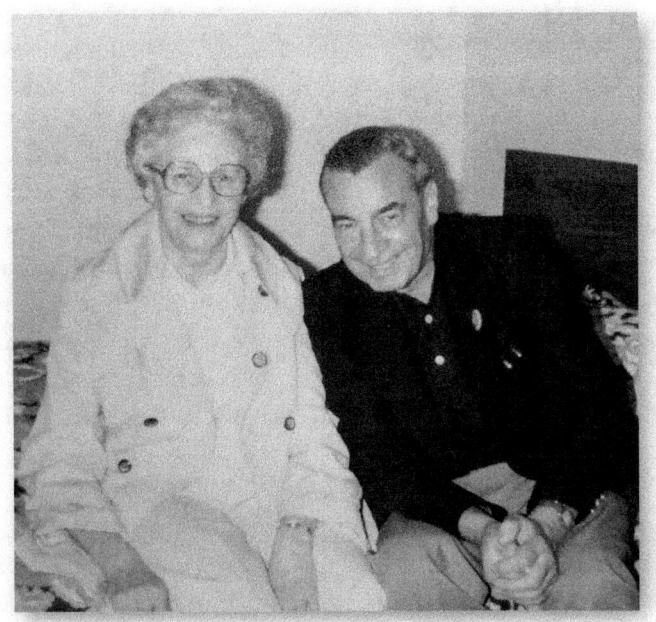

My parents, Mary and Harry Prenon, Philadelphia, PA, 1980

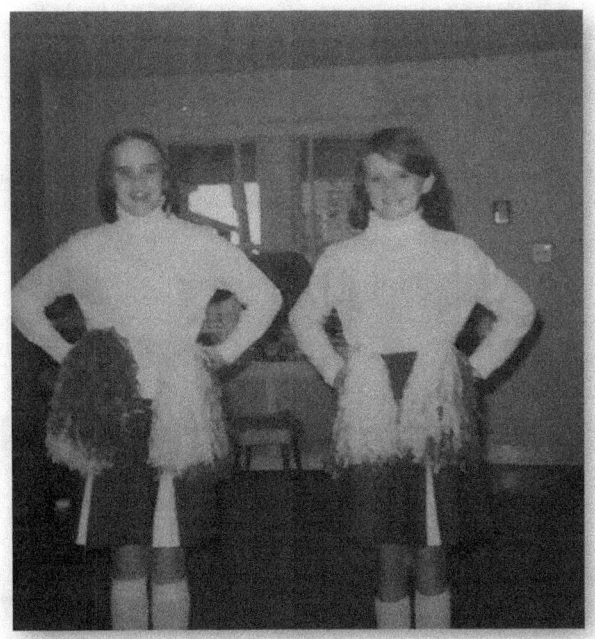

From left, Me and my friend Mary Liz as cheerleaders in Sixth
Grade at St. Charles School, Drexel Hill, PA, 1969

and my parents spent oodles of money on creams, ointments, pills, and even the occasional shot (ouch!).

During that time, I was also a dentist's dream. I lived for sweets. (Mom told me about the first time she let me try some chocolate. My eyes lit up, and I reached out both hands and said, "More." That behavior has continued to this day.) I had the misfortune of going to a local dentist who had attended school with all of the neighborhood parents. This madman was the go-to guy for the parents of all the local kids. He looked like the character Colonel Klink from the old TV show *Hogan's Heroes*. He didn't believe in numbing the tooth area before drilling, and years later my friends and I still had nightmares about being held down in the chair while the Frankenstein monster drilled our teeth and we screamed in pain. It was truly something out of the Dark Ages.

I had also been blessed with those awful metallic braces. I rarely smiled. One time, when my family was vacationing at the Jersey Shore with the Doughertys (the neighbors who had ten kids), Mary Liz and Jeanie, two of the Dougherty daughters, removed part of my braces when they became stuck on a candy apple. (Mom was not happy about that.)

By the time age sixteen rolled around, the braces had come off for good, and my skin had begun to clear up. Still a "skinny Minnie," I looked decent for both my junior and senior prom photos.

I entered college in 1975 and worked as a temp during the summers. The extra money I earned secured my spot in a summerhouse rental in Margate, New Jersey, with the women who would become my lifelong friends. Many a late night was spent imbibing too many beers and pizzas, but somehow my body was able to shrug off any extra weight—at least for a while.

After I graduated from college in 1979 and began working full time, my weight started to edge upward ever so slightly. (Note: with full-time employment, I was finally able to seek out a normal dentist, who not only used numbing medications but also called patients afterward to see how they were feeling!)

About my first job—after earning a BA in journalism from Temple University, and applying to every newspaper and advertising agency in the Philadelphia area, I landed a job as a secretary at an engineering firm. Apparently, I should have majored in welding. Still, I was happy to have a job after months of nothing. The former Pope John Paul had been visiting Philadelphia on the day I was hired, and Mom swore it was a true miracle. Eventually, the job morphed into a marketing-assistant position, although the salary was more like that of a scullery maid.

By my mid-twenties, the acne had disappeared, but then tiny fat rolls began to appear around my midsection. Being fairly young, though, it was pretty easy to get in shape rather quickly. Only a couple of times a week at the gym used to do it for me. (Little did I know that thirty years later, a couple of times a week would be just a warm-up.)

At the age of twenty-six, in 1983, I embarked on a major life change—I headed to New York to seek my fortune as a true journalist. In reality, I was offered a job as a technical writer for a computer software company. It wasn't my ideal job, but at least I'd be writing. (Hey, technical manuals can be very interesting!) At age twenty-nine I got married, and during my early thirties, the struggle to maintain a healthy weight became even harder. When I started to pack on the pounds, I tried many different kinds of fad diets, including those stupid liquid diets. By the end of the day, I was ready to eat my car. I can't remember how much I weighed then, but I do know that I was just about squeezing into a size fourteen.

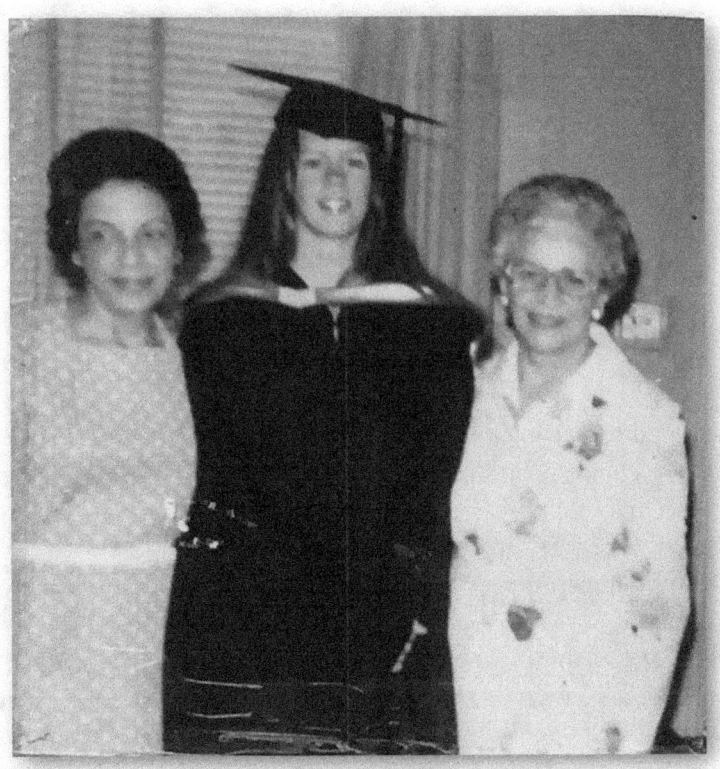

From left, "Aunt Tiny," Me and Mom at my college
graduation in Philadelphia, PA, 1979

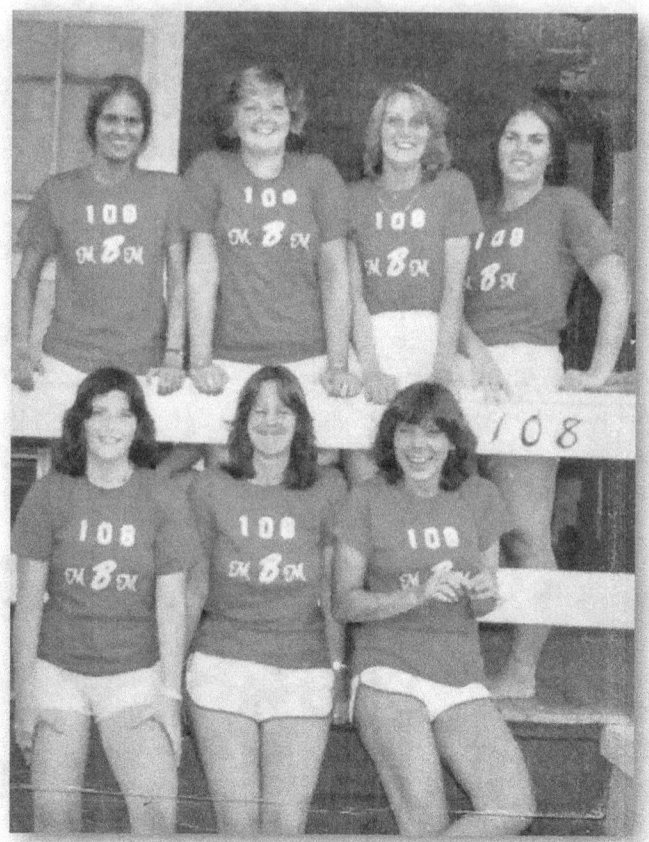

The Margate, NJ Crew, 1979
From left, (top row) Pam, Peggy, Mary Kay, and Terry S.
From left, (bottom row) Helen, Me, and Terry B.

Determined to put my journalism degree to work, I eventually left the computer software company and took a job at a local radio station as a news writer and anchor. It may sound exciting, but the job paid little more than minimum wage. I worked data entry at night to make ends meet. I later moved through two more radio stations before making a decent wage. Of course, my weight was still in "growth" mode.

One of the many things contributing to this "growth" was that fact that as a radio reporter, one would always be confronted with food while covering various events. Since we were all quite poor, we would stuff ourselves to the gills at any event where free food was abundant. Election nights were the best in terms of glomming free food. While the local village mayoral elections offered sandwiches and chips, the serious food was always served at Congressional election headquarters. If you were lucky enough to get assigned to a Congressional race, you could eat enough to fill your gut for three days.

Back at the radio station, ordinary days would turn to glorious ones when the sales department had their meetings. Afterward, they would send all of the leftover bagels to the newsroom. We would eat at least two helpings and save another two for the following day. (To this day, I still have a hard time turning down free food, despite the fact that I can now comfortably afford a bagel or sandwich.)

In 1991, at the age of thirty-four, a mini-miracle occurred. I lost a significant amount of weight and got down to an unbelievable 140 pounds! At that point, I had switched gears from news and found myself hosting a morning show on a rock music radio station in suburban New York City. One of our clients was a local hospital that was offering weight-loss programs. For advertising the program on my show, I got all their weight-loss counseling and medical advice for free, plus a talent fee each time I advertised the program live on the air. All I had to do was drop the weight. Pretty simple. And I did, because I wanted the money. I kept the weight off for about a year, but put it right back on again after my mother's death and my divorce. (Ironically, I think at 140 pounds I was too thin, because so many people kept asking me if I was OK. Rumors were swirling that I was somehow "very sick," and people were expecting my demise at any moment. When they started to see the weight returning, the general prognosis was that I would live!)

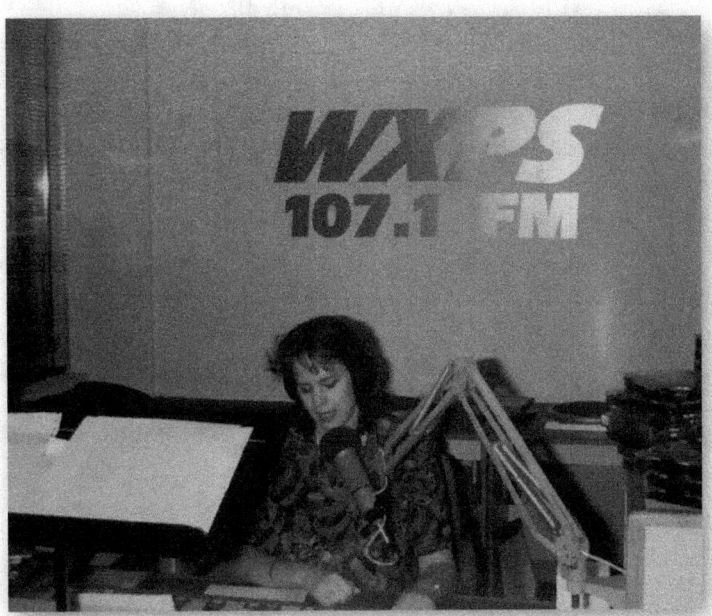

Me hosting the morning radio show on the now defunct WXPS in suburban New York City.

By 1998 though, at age forty-one, my girth had really gotten out of control. I had been working as a newspaper reporter, living way beyond my means in a beautiful new condo I'd recently purchased. I knew I'd have a tough time swinging the mortgage payments along with my car payment and other household expenses, but what the hell? I wasn't getting any younger. And with no kids to take care of, I could stretch to make ends meet.

Unfortunately, the stretching started to wear thin, and I had to do something to earn more money. I did some freelance writing and even sold cosmetics on the side, but it wasn't enough. I had been dutifully looking for another job, but most reporters' salaries were no better than what I was earning.

Desperate to earn more money, I made the unholy decision to transfer into the sales department at the newspaper. Now, there's nothing wrong with selling advertising space. It can be a very lucrative career if you have the stamina for it. Unfortunately, I didn't. After the first two weeks of acclimating myself to the new career, I realized I was in Hell. I hated it more than I hated my very first job at the age of sixteen—working in a hospital kitchen scraping garbage off the dinner plates of sick people for $1.80 an hour. To help ease the pain, I ate and ate and ate—candy bars, ice cream, potato chips, cookies—anything that would give me a moment's pleasure from that quagmire of corporate gobbledygook.

Soon I found that most of my clothes were too tight to wear, so I had to resort to buying skirts with lots of elastic. The beautiful formfitting dresses I had ordered earlier in the year couldn't even be zipped. I hated to get up in the morning, because I knew finding something to wear that fit was going to be struggle. Then I'd go to work and eat more. Finally, I made one of the smartest decisions of my life—I quit my job. I had nothing lined up and no real prospects, but I knew if I kept working there, I would lose my body and my mind.

I lived on freelance writing work and my savings for a while, and then landed a job with a local public relations/advertising agency. (Well, I didn't "land" it like, "Alikazam...here's a job." I knew the people there from writing stories about many of their clients while I was at the newspaper. Yes, it *does* help to know the right people.) Things were looking up, and I could finally concentrate on getting back in shape. A new job—a new lease on life.

That was wishful thinking. The reality is, I continued to gain weight, and while I did exercise, it apparently wasn't enough. I didn't enjoy going to the gym, and my new job required me to attend a lot of events—and where there are events, there's lots of food.

I continued to eat way too much—at events, in the office, and at home. What got me back on track, for at least a little while, was a horrific gall bladder attack. It was 2003, and at the age of forty-five I got down to 175 pounds. The pain from the gallstone was so bad that I could not eat until I was full (more on this later). It took me a relatively short time—maybe a couple of months—to drop about fifteen pounds, simply because I wanted to avoid pain. After an operation to remove the gallstone, I managed to keep the weight off for a while. Of course, I eventually gained it all back— and more. I obviously continued to reward myself for surviving the operation. I had fallen into the yo-yo trap once again.

Toward the end of my forties, I hit menopause, which in itself is a weight changer. Everyone says dropping the tonnage after you hit menopause is much harder, and, yes, it's true. You have to work twice as hard as you did in your thirties and probably three times as hard as you did in your twenties.

At age forty-eight, I had another life-changing situation that somehow translated to weight gain. I completely switched careers. Stressed out by the demanding grind of the ad agency, I left to attend esthetician school so that I could do facials in a spa. One of my former clients at the ad agency was a high-end spa in the Berkshires in western Massachusetts, and I loved the atmosphere. I decided that's what I wanted, and, yes, I was the oldest student in the class.

I graduated from the six-month program, took the New York State boards, got my license, and began working at a couple of spas. The work was wonderful and peaceful, but I began stressing about not making enough money again. So, I ended up back at the ad agency a few days a week and "spa-ing" the other days. The good news was, the arrangement worked well. The bad news—I didn't get any thinner.

Then I hit my fifties, when getting in shape is an entirely new ball game. It seemed like dropping the weight and getting in shape would be impossible. At age fifty-three, I took a new job as director of communications at a regional New York Realtor association. (Ironically, newspaper ad sales is part of my job now, and I actually like it. Who knew?) Thinking again that a new career would help to get the scale moving south, I had a few successes, but a lot more setbacks. In fact, it would be seven long, hard years before I finally achieved my weight goal.

A year before, in 2009, I had also started my own spa and was doing facials and reflexology on the weekends. I have continued to operate my little spa since that time but have cut back on the amount of time dedicated to it. Offering a couple of facials on the weekend is enjoyable and is great "mad money" as well!

I just recently turned sixty and I have to tell you, that number is still really freaking me out. All those fun times in Margate, New Jersey, seem like yesterday! What the hell happened? Anyhow, my new motto now is, "Any day above ground is a good one!"

So in a nutshell, that's my story of how I went from skinny to not so "thinny" over the years. No matter what size you are, laughing is so important. It's kept me sane—or relatively sane—for those years when I was really struggling and frustrated. It also beats the hell out of crying and feeling sorry for yourself.

Now, before moving on to what to do to fix the problem, let's talk about what *not* to do in the next chapter.

CHAPTER 2
Avoiding Fad Diets and Negative Body Image

"Diet" is another word that should be banned, along with the phrase "weight loss." No one should ever be "on a diet." Instead, we should say we're going to make healthier choices when eating. Yeah, right. That's a lot easier said than done.

Almost every day we're bombarded with messages about how easy and fun it is to get in shape and "lose weight." Pick up any magazine, and you're bound to see that phrase in screaming headlines—"Lose Weight in Two Hours," "Lose Weight and Solve the National Debt," "Lose Weight and Conquer the World." SHADDAP already! Please! "Lose weight" is simply the most stupid, ridiculous, frustrating, irritating, and infuriating phrase in the English language. I truly believe that phrase is the downfall of anyone who is trying to go from flabby to firm.

Think about it. When you say you "lost" something, isn't it assumed that you want to find it again, like, "I lost my keys" or "I lost my wallet"? Doesn't it imply that you didn't intend to misplace anything? Ergo, doesn't it stand to reason that if you "lost" weight, you simply misplaced it and will find it again sooner or later? "Hmmm...I lost twenty pounds. Where the hell could they have gone?" And before you know it, you find them again. "Yikes! Here they are in my right butt cheek!"

Eating healthy and exercising takes time and planning. Getting to your goal weight or fitness level doesn't happen overnight. And if you're lazy like me, it can be a huge turnoff. Years ago when I was driving to work one day, I saw a poster on a telephone pole that was guaranteeing a weight loss of thirty pounds in thirty days. I considered calling the 800 number listed, but then I realized that losing so much weight in one month would probably require a little help from a chainsaw. After all, the ad didn't say you'd be *alive* at the end of thirty days.

There are so many fads out there that it's difficult to know what's real and what's fake. The rule of thumb I've learned to follow is that if it sounds too good to be true, it probably is. There are pills, juices, teas, chewy bars, and tablets, plus weird combinations of food. There are low-carb, low-fat, low-sugar, low-sodium, high-protein, and liquid-only diets, and scads of others on the market. And guess what—most of them are waiting to separate you from your money.

Look at the supermarket tabloids. I recently saw an ad in one for another "miracle" diet that will allegedly enable you to shed nine pounds in five days. Sure, I believe it. It's furniture polish. Drink some with dinner and become violently ill and unable to eat for five days. Voilà! There's your weight loss.

I even tried hypnosis, but it didn't work for me. I'm naturally skeptical and was afraid that I'd end up walking down Main Street in a duck suit during rush hour.

I have to admit that years ago I did succumb to many—and I mean many—fad diets. I did the liquids, the protein bars, the grapefruit, the soup, and many other really stupid eating plans. One in particular was promoted by one of those weight-loss centers that I think are now out of business—at least in New York. The best part was that the center I chose to go to was right smack inbetween a Boston Market and a pastry shop. Seriously, you can't make this stuff up.

At any rate, I was instructed to eat next to nothing, and I could have two of their "protein bars" a day. Of course, there was no nutritional information on the alleged protein bars, so they were probably loaded with sugar and carbs. What I found really strange, though, was that there was no mention of exercising. Needless to say, I didn't lose an ounce. One week I did work out like hell with walking and aerobics classes, and I managed to lose a couple of pounds. The "trained specialist" at the center told me that exercising was OK, but what would really work was their insane "diet." The final straw was when I was told my goal weight should be 135 pounds. Excuse me? I politely told the woman that if I ever did get to 135 pounds, I would probably have to be hospitalized for malnutrition and starvation. That was the last time I ever set foot in that hellhole.

Of course, there are lots of TV ads for weight-loss schemes, especially for "fat" pills. These pills allegedly flush the fat out of your system after you eat. Yeah, sounds great, with one little minor side effect—"inability to control bowel movements." I don't know about you, but that's something I don't want to play around with. How's that going to go over in the office? Right in the middle of a presentation—bawoosh! "Oops...sorry about that mess." Yeah, I don't *think* so.

Here's one for the "How stupid are you to fall for this crap?" commercials. While sweating and panting like a puma at the gym one day, one of those "You can really look this good!" infomercials came on the TV. They were hawking an "ab chair," not to be confused with the now-unpopular "ab roller." Here's the deal. You sit in this special ergonomically correct chair and push side to side and back to front and voilà! Within a few days you have abs of steel. And if that's not enough to convince you, hey—this handy dandy chair "even folds away for convenient storage." OK, ready for the price tag? $180! Yep, $180 to do the same exact thing you could do yourself on the floor. In fact, you'll get an even better workout if you do it yourself, but there's a sucker out there every minute who will slap down any amount of money for a miracle cure. I think I'll invent the Miracle Butt Shaper. It'll be a child's booster seat that you try to squeeze your cheeks into. I think it will retail for $225, plus tax.

In addition to crazy diets and overpriced exercise equipment, we're also barraged by catalogs selling tummy control panties, control-top pantyhose, and girdles. Now, these are not like Mom's girdles, mind you. These are the new "I Can't Believe It's a Girdle" girdles. (Help! I can't believe I'm thinking of buying one!) You can get the one that flattens just the tummy, or you can go for the gusto and get the one that soothes the hips and thighs as well. At the end of the day, you simply remove it and explode.

The world is trying to change its attitude about what constitutes a "healthy body," but many magazine covers still show extremely skinny women who are touted as being healthy. News bulletin—a curvy woman can be healthy! You don't have to have a completely flat stomach, twig-like legs, and tiny boobs to be healthy.

I recently read an article about a plus-size model who was five feet seven inches and weighed 145 pounds. Huh? Plus size? Who the hell comes up with that crap, some anorexic moron? How can a normal-sized (or, in this case, thin) person be considered a plus size? Gimme a break. If I ever find the nitwits who developed those criteria, I will personally stick a head of romaine lettuce up their butts.

Many women have a hard enough time with their body image, and when they're trying to get fit, the last thing in the world they want to see is one of those damn Victoria's Secret catalogs chock full of skinny women in skimpy outfits. I read some-where that the average size of the Victoria's Secret models is 4. Who the hell wears a size 4, a gnome? Maybe that's the secret Victoria's been keeping all these years—nobody wears a damn size four.

Men always want us to buy something from this catalog, too. What, do they think we're going to look like the model when we put it on? Men are so full of crap. They say stuff like, "Oh, honey, I can just picture how you'll look in this." And I reply, "Oh, in that case, let me tell you. I'll look fat!"

But then again, maybe that's not true. As the old saying goes, "beauty is in the eye of the beholder." In fact, my absolute favorite episode of *The Twilight Zone* is "Eye of the Beholder." If you haven't seen it, beg, borrow, or steal a recording of it. It's a must-watch episode. The story is about a woman who longs to be beautiful and the team of plastic surgeons who have been committed over the years to making that happen. Throughout the episode, they never allow you to get a good look at anyone's face, but you assume that the doctors are normal-looking people and that the woman is some grotesque monster. After her final operation, one of the doctors recoils in horror and shouts, "No change!" The woman is diminished to tears and anguish. However, when the camera finally shows the woman, she's as beautiful as a movie star, and the people who are supposed to be normal are actually hideous. In their world, our perception of beauty is ugliness and vice versa. After watching this episode, when I looked down at my flabby body with cottage cheese thighs and ham hock arms, I realized that in some other world, I was incredibly fit, sexy, and hot, while lingerie models and centerfolds were disgusting and frumpy. The only problem was, how could I possibly get to that other world?

Sometimes, all we need to help improve our body image is a new outfit or a new bra. The fact is, as we age, our body parts begin to droop. My boobs had long ago ventured on the journey south, but I never did anything about it. I hated underwire bras and refused to wear them. I didn't see it as a big problem, but, occasionally, it did look like I had three or four boobs. I guess everything got mashed together. Still, that wasn't enough to make me change my "no underwire bras" policy.

Enter my gay co-worker. At my current job at the Realtor association, Gary is our MLS (Multiple Listing Service) director, as well as our designated party planner. Gary is never one to hold back his opinions, and after knowing him for a few years, he felt very comfortable telling me that my "girls" were drooping.

One day, he called me and my coworker, Emily, into his office, demanding that Emily take me to Nordstrom's and help me find a new bra. (Our office is across the street from a very chic mall.) Like two doe-eyed bobbleheads, we agreed. Off we went to the lingerie department of Nordstrom's, where the corsetiere (a.k.a. "bra fitter") measured us both and then brought in a myriad of boulder-holders for us to try on. Then the hijinks ensued.

Emily and I began trying the underwire wonders on our heads, and in a short time we had the entire dressing room full of women laughing their asses off. The corsetiere came in shortly afterward, explaining that, yes, the garment may feel a little different if one has never worn an underwire bra before—where it's supposed to be worn, that is. A little different? I felt like a middle-aged Viking woman suiting up to go into battle. Ergo, the nickname "Helga" was given to the wretched brassiere.

After Emily and I composed ourselves, we purchased our respective "Helgas" and headed back to the office. I walked past Gary's office to see if he noticed the new purchase, and there he was, smiling and clapping. Mind you, if he had been a straight man talking about my droopage, he would have been slapped with a sexual harassment lawsuit. But gay men are usually right on the money when it comes to fashion. I know that sounds cliché, but it's true. In fact, we often now refer to Gary as "Mr. Blackwell."

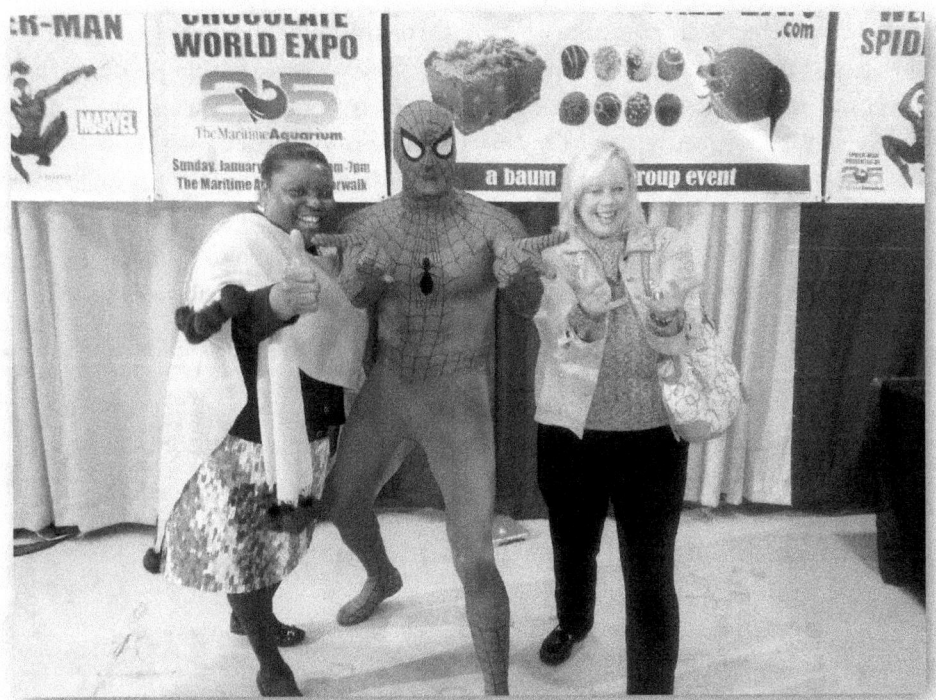

From left, Emily and Me with Spiderman at the Chocolate Festival in White Plains, NY, 2013

The first few weeks with the underwire bra were torturous. I ripped the thing off as soon as I got home. Eventually, though, I got used to it and actually liked the way I looked. It lifted the "girls" away from my stomach, so it gave the appearance that I had become thinner.

For so many years I dealt with a negative body image, and I can tell you now that it was a colossal waste of my time and energy. I was so concerned about my outward appearance that it almost started to take away from who I really was on the inside. Fortunately, I was able to stop and say, "Wait a minute, this is bullshit!"

First of all, no one has a perfect body—except maybe newborns. We all have something, or in my case, many things, we don't like about our bodies. And while we all want to look good and be healthier, we have to realize that it can be a very long journey. So why not make the journey fun?

While you're working on getting healthy, it's just as important to concentrate on your inner beauty and let that shine through. None of us are defined by our flesh. It's our smiles, our laughter, and our love of life that create our unique personalities. Don't ever let images of seemingly "perfect" bodies attack your self-esteem. So you may look a little different—so what? You are who you are on the inside and no one can ever take that away from you. Sure, you can work toward a goal, but while you're doing that, never put yourself down or let others put you down. And if someone is ever rude or judgmental, please feel free to use my motto, "Go screw yourself!"

The bottom line is that—in my experience—there is no "miracle" diet, pill, food, drink, or exercise product that takes weight off at the speed of light. In my case, the road to healthy living has been paved with a lot of crap that didn't work. Let me reiterate—making healthy food choices and committing to regular exercise truly sucks, but once you realize that and stick with it anyway, you will start to see and feel the difference in your body and mind. I guarantee that changing the way you eat and move will make you a hundred times happier than pizza and ice cream do. In the upcoming chapters, I'll explain how to do it without spiraling into complete madness.

How I Avoid Fads and Negative Body Image

1. Switch the TV channel whenever you see a weight-loss commercial.
2. Switch the radio station if you hear a weight-loss commercial.
3. Pick up a supermarket tabloid with screaming headlines about cellulite on a supposedly skinny movie star or model. Realize they are just like us.
4. View magazine covers with a grain of salt. Most of the photos are airbrushed.
5. Look at yourself in the mirror and smile (although many times I just laugh). Seriously, look beyond your body, and see your inner beauty. It's definitely there.

CHAPTER 3

Motivating Yourself (and Maintaining Your Sanity)

OK, so before we delve into our new phase of eating healthy and exercising, we have to be motivated. But why? Why can't we just get up and do it? We don't need motivation to go to the bathroom, take a shower or brush our teeth—we do these things because otherwise, we'd stink. For some reason, though, we need motivation to eat healthy and exercise. It could be that those two things have become unnatural in today's hectic world. In fact, it *is* easier to grab some fast food than to prepare a whole dinner. It's also easier to sit and check your e-mail on your tablet or watch TV than to put your body through a workout routine.

Now that we've established that we *do* need motivation to live healthy, how do we get that motivation? I've tried many different motivational techniques over the years. I've listened to motivational tapes, read inspirational books, and kept up-to-date with the latest health magazines. The only motivation I ever got was to eat chips while listening or reading.

I've also attended motivational seminars. At one in particular, attendees were led to believe that their problems stemmed from a rotten self-image. Apparently, I had been sabotaging myself every time I referred to myself in derogatory terms, like "bubble butt" or "lard ass." The new objective was to program my subconscious mind into thinking of myself as a winner. While it's unrealistic to say I had already achieved my goals when I clearly hadn't, I did try to reprogram my way of thinking. All night long, I'd tell myself that I *am* the kind of person who likes to work out, no matter how tired or grumpy I feel. I *am* the kind of person who sticks to her fitness goals, no matter how depressed I am about my current weight. I *am* the kind of person who likes to eat healthy.

The problem is, I don't believe I *am* a very programmable person. I guess that's why religious cults never had an effect on me. (It could also be that I'm notoriously cheap.) Mom never worried about me running off to join a cult. Her reflections on the subject were very clear: "The first time they ask you for a dime, you'll be running out the door." True, all true.

I once had the opportunity to see a semi-famous motivational speaker. At the ad agency where I'd worked, one of our clients—a major residential real estate firm in suburban New York City—held its annual awards luncheon at a fashionable catering hall. The tables were beautifully appointed with flowers, glistening glassware, and fine silver. Each table was also adorned with two plates of cheeses and fruit—a nice beginning course.

After everyone was seated, I listened happily through the introductory speeches and looked forward to what I thought would be a motivating thirty-minute keynote address. Wrong! I knew I was in trouble when this "noted author" informed the audience at the start that he'd be speaking for the next hour or so. Huh? Everyone at my table and the surrounding tables gasped, looked at each other in bewilderment, and slowly settled in for a long winter's nap. On and on he went. Shakespeare said it best— "much ado about nothing." After about a half hour, people started shifting uncomfortably in their chairs, then passing around the cheese plates.

This guy didn't let up for a minute, jumping from topic to topic like he was playing leap frog. From ancient philosophers whose names I can't pronounce, to a young child in tenth century Nepal, to Mother Theresa and the homeless. Yes, the homeless— at a real estate luncheon celebrating a multibillion-dollar year. Hello? Then this so-called "motivational speaker" threw in something about not worrying about money or material possessions. Meanwhile, his staff members were out in the lobby hawking his books and tapes for twenty-five dollars a pop.

After about an hour and several rounds of the cheese plates, my stomach began to growl and my patience wore thin. Many people left their seats on the pretext of going to the bathroom, and I, of course, was among them. A small crowd quickly gathered in the lobby, and we took turns peeking through the door to see if the horror show was over yet. Finally, after an hour and forty minutes, he decided to pack it in. I returned to my table with the others en masse, hungry as a lion in a barren wasteland.

For almost two hours, I had to rely on cheese and grapes to get through that nightmare. While the lunch of crab salad we were eventually served was delicious, my stomach sought much more after that diatribe. On the way back to the office, I was forced to make an emergency detour to McDonald's.

I once tried motivating myself to exercise by treating it like a job. After all, I thought, if I stayed in bed all day and didn't go to work, I'd soon find myself living in a cardboard box underneath the New York State Thruway. Unfortunately, that didn't pan out well, because after putting in a full day of work, the last thing I wanted to do was go to another "job."

I even tried to get motivated by hanging up photos of myself when I was thin (at age eighteen) and of a thin, fit woman. It didn't work. I knew I'd never be eighteen again, and I ended up just being jealous of the thin, fit woman.

I also tried hanging a dress and a pair of pants that no longer fit on the outside of my closet door. That way I'd see them every morning when I got up and be motivated to fit into them again. Nope. I decided the clothes were out of style and threw them out.

I thought wanting to look great for a wedding or some other big event would be a good motivator. But, I ultimately reasoned that everyone is usually so drunk at those things, they wouldn't remember what I looked like anyway.

One really good motivator was a gallstone. It started in 2003, at the age of forty-six, when I experienced excruciating stomach pain. For those of you who have had it, you know what I'm talking about. For those who haven't, imagine a monster's hand wrapped around your stomach, squeezing the hell out of it, and then the monster's hand moves around to your back and starts squeezing there, too. Now maybe you can understand why I'd do anything—even eat right—to avoid that pain.

After trying to get motivated from all of that "happy talk" crap, the fear of pain won out. I was so terrified of having another gall bladder attack that I started to avoid any type of fatty foods that would trigger one. Even eating too much healthy food could trigger an attack—apparently, "Gally" didn't like a full stomach. As a result, I stopped eating just short of feeling full. Sure, I was a little hungry, but I'd rather deal with hunger pains than a gallstone attack.

The gallstone motivation worked very well, and I got down to 175 pounds. However, after the gallstone was removed, the surgeon told me I could eat whatever I wanted, and I eagerly followed his advice. Basically, I went ape shit from Thanksgiving to the end of January. I had discovered a newfound freedom of eating junk foods without pain. As for the gallstone, I still have it displayed in a cute little case on my desk in my home office. I'd hoped for a while that it would remotivate me, but without the pain, the motivation was gone. I even jokingly suggested that the surgeon put the stone back in. Very sick, I know.

With the weight gain came new problems—high blood pressure and high choles-terol. My primary care doctor often suggested that I eat healthier and exercise so she wouldn't have to prescribe medications. I tried, but not hard enough. My laziness and lack of focus resulted in getting prescriptions for both blood pressure and cholesterol medications.

At age fifty-three, the fear of an untimely death did prove to be a bit more moti-vating. About a month after starting my new job as the communications director for a Realtor association, I attended a sales award function. The food was mediocre, but I was damn hungry, so I began to inhale the fatty, salty, fried crap. One of my colleagues joked that Alpo had catered the affair.

Later that night, my heart felt like it was drag racing, and I ended up going to the ER at the local hospital. After an EKG, blood tests, and chest x-rays, they found noth-ing wrong. My theory was that my racing heart was caused by a combination of the junk I ate plus the blood pressure medication I had been on for a while, which had been linked to irregular heartbeats.

The next day, I went to my primary care doctor, had another EKG, and then went through the litany of heart checks: heart monitor, echocardiogram, stress test, and more blood work. Again, nothing was wrong. The end result was a change in my blood pres-sure medication and the introduction of my cardiologist, who I will refer to as "Dr. K."

Now, I had major motivation. Not necessarily because I wanted a long, healthy life after that heart scare, but because Dr. K told me I was fat. Well, he didn't actually use the "F" word—he told me I was "heavy." In fact, his exact words were, "Well, you *are* heavy, but you're not the heaviest person I've ever seen." I couldn't believe it! No one had ever said anything like that to me before in my life—probably for fear of being bludgeoned to death.

At first, I wanted to strangle Dr. K with my bare hands. Didn't he realize that totally pissing off a menopausal woman was *not* a good thing? Then I thought, "So, I'm not the heaviest person you've ever seen? What, was there a sumo wrestler in here right before me?" I wanted to say this and more, but I was speechless. Then I thought about suing him for slander or emotional distress.

Instead, I just stood there, making lame promises to exercise more and eat health-ier. All the while, I was in disbelief that he had told me I was heavy. Look, it's not like I didn't already know I was overweight, and I'm sure lots of people thought I was too, but no one had ever dared to tell me that. After I left his office, I felt a mixture of emo-tions. The thing is, Dr. K is a very good physician and someone who really cares about his patients. He has a friendly demeanor and I knew he didn't intend to be hurtful, but his comments cut through me like a butcher knife.

As soon as I left his office, I didn't know whether to cry or scream. I went for the screaming first. I called my best friend, Madam, and went into a tirade about what this "awful man" had said to me. We secretly plotted to kidnap him and stuff him with junk food until he was 500 pounds. Later, I went for the crying, but after I finished I started to get really angry. I was angry with Dr. K for being truthful, but I was even angrier with myself for letting things get out of control. "I'll show him who was heavy," I thought. "I'll eat nothing but bean sprouts and exercise every day for hours, and then I'll show him."

Again, this was easier said than done. Soon afterward, I ran into Dr. K at a gym I had joined earlier in the year. (More about gyms and health clubs in the next chapter). I was looking particularly dumpy that day and was sweating profusely after hoisting barbells and wrestling with some of the weight machines. Out of the corner of my eye, I saw a familiar face and then heard, "Hi, Mary, glad to see you're working out." Apparently, Dr. K was also a member of this gym, but I jokingly asked him if he was checking up on me to make sure I was exercising. Over the next few days I was very careful about what I ate for fear he would spring out of some corner and snatch a cheeseburger from my hand.

Looking back now, his comment may have been the best thing that anyone has ever said to me. Since that time, I did have more incidents of irregular heartbeat, or atrial fibrillation (a.k.a. "AFib"). The next time was in 2014, at age fifty-seven. I had been working in the yard all day, drinking very little water, and then ordered a big Indian food dinner (that was probably loaded with sodium). Fortunately, my heart corrected itself in a couple of hours.

Then in late October 2015 I had my first all-nighter with AFib. Since I had gone to the gym earlier than evening, I told myself it was OK to have a large piece of buffalo chicken pizza for dinner. Unfortunately, I didn't drink enough water while eating the pizza, and then followed it up with a bag of popcorn. Shortly afterward, the band started playing in my chest. There was no pain, no shortness of breath, and no dizziness, just a weird feeling of a drum beating way out of time.

I spent the night in the ER of my local hospital, and miraculously, as the cardiologist was preparing to shock my heart back into rhythm, it corrected on its own. The running joke at the hospital is that once people see the cardiologist, they get so freaked out that their hearts jolt back into normal behavior. Whatever it was, I was lucky.

Ironically, it was the same hospital where I had been working out that day. Early in 2015, I learned from a neighbor that the hospital had a Wellness Club that was open to the public. Apparently, it had been there for years, but I never knew about it. I joined, and it has been the best thing that ever happened to me.

For many years, I hated going to the gym because most gyms are big, impersonal places where you feel like a number instead of a person. I'd find a new gym and be very enthusiastic in the beginning, but after dealing with overcrowded conditions and lack of friendliness, I'd lose interest quickly. Then it became a chore—"I have to go to the gym"—and no one likes chores.

The Wellness Club is small and has a friendly staff. The classes are also small, and a personal trainer is on hand at all times to help with anything. Best of all, they have a computer to track your workouts, and every time you go, you earn fitness points. You can achieve different fitness levels, and each month, your name goes up on the bulletin board showing your current fitness level. Yes, it's like school, but it is motivating because it keeps you striving to get to the next level.

I especially like this place because it's never crowded, and most of its members are seniors. (Technically, I'm a senior now that I'm over fifty-five, but I don't think I've accepted that yet.) There are no twentysomethings running around in designer gym gear or making grunting noises while hoisting weights. The people at the front desk know me by name and take time to stop and chat. I've also gotten to know some of the other members.

I truly believe that finding the right place and the right activity that works for you is half the battle of dropping the tonnage and getting in shape. You don't have to join a gym. Walking outside is great exercise, and in the cold weather, head to the local mall and walk indoors.

If you view exercise as something you have to do it's not going to work. You have to turn it into something you want to do.

As I've said, I tried the positive motivation of feeling good about myself and had the negative motivation of the grim reaper creeping closely behind me. I've tried setting goals to be a certain weight, to fit into certain clothes by a specific date (e.g., the first day of summer), and to get in shape for weddings and other special occasions. None of that worked (with the exception, of course, of the gall bladder operation, and there the motivation was severe pain).

So what's the final answer? Here it is plain and simple—don't think too much. I wasted so much time trying to motivate myself instead of just doing what I had to do. It's literally taken me nineteen years to discover that there's no secret formula for motivation—everyone is different, and what works for one person may not work for someone else.

Here's what I do know—find what works for *you*. This may take some time, as it did for me. (OK, a lot of time.) But once you do find what works—a big gym, a small gym, no gym, playing sports, walking outside, swimming, biking, and so forth—you'll be motivated to do it and to stick with it.

And when you like the type of exercise you're doing and start seeing results, you'll be naturally inclined to make healthier eating choices, because you won't want to wreck what you've accomplished.

In the next chapter, we'll talk about how to keep those workouts going, especially when you're tired or lazy—as is the story of my life!

What Motivates Me

1. Chatting with people I've met at the Wellness Club and being able to commiserate with them while working out.
2. Being able to fit into clothes I haven't worn in years
3. Feeling less of a jiggle in my arms, legs, and butt.
4. Generally feeling better both physically and emotionally.
5. Being complimented about the way I look.
6. Normal blood pressure and cholesterol numbers.
7. A smile instead of a scowl on my cardiologist's face.
8. The fear of death (that's always a good one!).

CHAPTER 4

Working in Those Workouts (Even When the Couch is Calling)

Now that you're motivated and you've hopefully found the type of exercise that works for you, how do you stay committed to it?

I have to admit that sometimes I am damn sick and tired of walking, kicking, cycling, and heaving barbells every day just so I can look like a normal human being instead of a human beach ball. I've been at this thing my life entire life and, unfortunately, the big bottom (no pun intended) line is—this is the way it's going to be until they come up with a "body-in-a-bottle." Why? Because if we don't exercise, we're screwed with stuff like lower back pain, arthritis, heart disease, cancer, and God knows what else.

I assure you that I do not get up every day and say, "Wow, I can't wait to do the elliptical machine and some crunches!" I do make it a point to go to the gym almost every day after work, even though some days I crawl back to the locker room, sweating like an old mare that finished last in the Kentucky Derby.

Nothing comes easy. Sure, there are people who can eat a fifteen-course meal every night, never exercise, and never gain an ounce. They are the minority in this world. In fact, I don't believe those people are human. I bet they never sleep either. Some extra-terrestrials don't need sleep.

As I've said before, working out doesn't necessarily mean you have to join a gym. Some fitness centers can be very intimidating. I can't tell you how many gyms I've joined and then gotten sick of them in just a few months. I'd take a week or two off, and then eventually go back to get my "money's worth."

I've tried high-end gyms, but couldn't keep up with the designer workout clothes. In one high-end gym, a very thin woman in a fabulous outfit of matching pants and top was on the elliptical machine next to mine. While I was huffing and puffing, she was going a mile a minute. I mean, her feet were moving so fast, she reminded me of Fred Flintstone starting the family car. I didn't think human begins could move so fast. "Probably another extraterrestrial," I thought.

Another problem with the high-end fitness centers was that most of the people there were already fit. I was the "before" photo in a sea of "after" photos. Some of the women wore full makeup, and they would smile and toss their hair while effortlessly climbing the Stairmaster. Eventually, a hulking man would approach them. The only guys who might approach me at one of these gyms would be plastic surgeons or pharmaceutical salesmen hawking the latest cellulite cream.

One night I overheard some twentysomethings in the gym talking about how someone they knew had to take it easy and couldn't do everything he used to because "he's not that young anymore." I figured they were talking about someone who was maybe seventy years old or more. Then I heard one of the women say the punch line, and I almost kerplotzed—"Yeah, you know, he's almost forty now." Almost forty? That's what they considered "getting old"! They would have definitely put me out to pasture.

I've also tried cheap gyms, but couldn't deal with the crowds. If I have to wait for a treadmill, it's not worth it. Plus, it's been my experience that the cheap gyms usually have lots of broken equipment, or machines that don't work well.

One time, at one of those "bargain" gyms, I had a minicrisis when my feet somehow got stuck in the rowing machine. Before starting, I had tightened the straps on the foot holders to make sure I didn't bob up and down. When I couldn't get my feet out of the foot holders, panic set in. Cautiously, I looked around to make sure no one could see me frantically fidgeting. Not only were my feet immobile, but I couldn't seem to loosen the straps either. After flailing around for a few minutes, I considered removing my sneakers and then trying to pry them loose. Fortunately, my fidgeting paid off and, one-by-one, my feet emerged from the foot holders. Since then, I have avoided the rowing machines.

Some gyms—both high end and low end—also have lots of mirrors and huge windows, which can be frightening. The last thing I wanted to see was my fat gut swaying back and forth right in front of me. One gym had huge windows overlooking the parking lot of the entire shopping center. The problem was that the backs of the treadmills were facing the windows so that everyone walking by could see people's butt cheeks flopping up and down.

I've also spent countless dollars on personal trainers. My theory was that if I threw a lot of money at my weight problem, it would surely be resolved. Looking back, I wouldn't say that I'd wasted the money. In fact, it was money well spent, but I didn't keep up the routine. I was lazy.

One of my trainers was a petite dynamo named C.J., who I later affectionately dubbed "C.J. the Torturer." This woman used to work me so hard, I often thought about making funeral arrangements for myself. Her mantra, which I still use today, was "Suck it up!"

When I'd arrive for my training session, she would point to the elliptical machine and say, "Twenty minutes." Each session, she'd increase the weights I had been using on both my arms and legs. At one point, I checked to see if my arm was still in its socket. If I threatened not to show up one day, C.J. would simply say, "I know where you live, and I'll come and get you."

With C.J.'s help, I did manage to drop some pounds, but, unfortunately, she ended up moving to California. I tried other trainers after that, but none were as good or as tough as C.J.

If you like to dance, that's a great workout. I love dancing, and I have my wild and crazy neighbor and friend, JoEllen, to thank for getting me back into this really fun form of exercise. We are now part of a motley cast of characters who meet almost every weekend to listen to a local band and tap our toes. Hey, girls just want to have fun, even if the girls are now in their fifties and sixties.

When I was in my twenties, my friends and I would get ready to go out at nine or ten o'clock at night. As we would enter a place, all of the "old people" would be leaving. We couldn't believe anyone would be going home so early and vowed to never let that happen to us. Well, fast forward thirty years and here we are, going out at seven o'clock for bands that start playing at seven thirty or eight, and then heading home by ten thirty or eleven. Sometimes, when my friends and I are visiting the New Jersey Shore or Cape Cod, Massachusetts, we go out even earlier, like four o'clock, to catch afternoon bands. By nine o'clock, we're spent. Some bands don't start until ten o'clock, and that's too late for us. Yep, we're definitely the "old people" now.

As I said before, walking is wonderful exercise that you can do just about anywhere. My neighborhood doesn't have sidewalks (it's a bit rural), so I usually go to parks, walking trails, or even the local high school track to walk. During the workday, I also use part of my lunch hour to walk outside. My friend and co-worker Leah and I do laps around the parking lot at lunch. Bring your phone to track your steps or invest in a "Fitbit" watch.

The weather can sometimes be a detriment to exercising outdoors. If there's a blizzard, it can be dangerous. If it's snowing lightly, however, you could get exercise by shoveling, building a snowman, or throwing snowballs at trees. In the summer, exercising in extreme heat can be harmful. God, how I detest the heat. When I was a child,

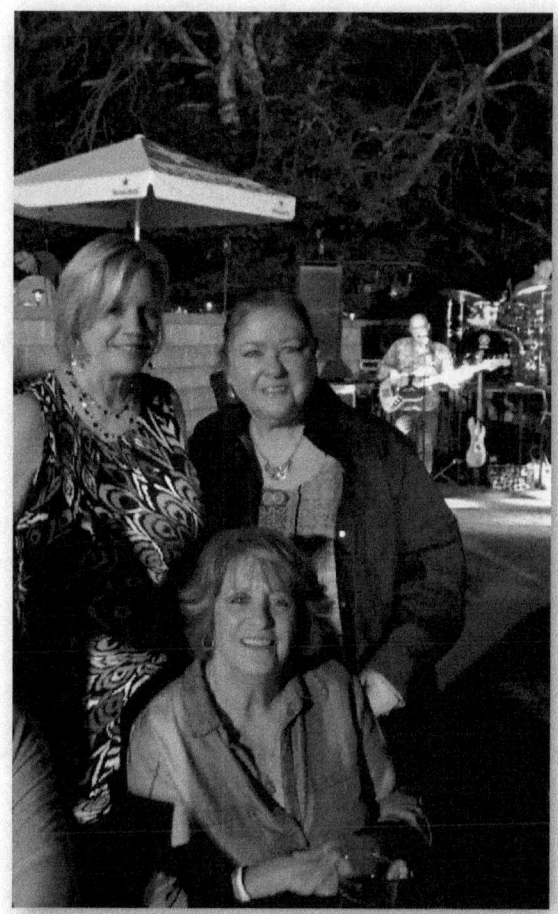

From left, Me, JoEllen and Gail (seated) out for a night of
dancing in Mahopac, NY, 2016

my parents were very concerned about conserving energy and saving money, and it was a major decision for them to turn on the air-conditioner (this is long before the days of central air). They would often try to convince me that the air conditioner was unnecessary because there was a "nice breeze," to which I would respond, "Where? Nome, Alaska?"

My mother would then use her famous line, "If you think it's hot here, just wait until you get to Purgatory." For those who are not of the Christian faith, Purgatory is a kind of "way station" between Heaven and Hell. Only the truly holy, like Mother Theresa and the guy who invented air-conditioning, get right into Heaven. The truly wicked, like murderers or manufacturers of size zero clothing, go straight to Hell. The rest of us slobs are going to Purgatory. No one knows how long you have to stay there. It could be days, months, or even years. The only thing we do know (according to my mother) is that it is damn hot in Purgatory. (This, however, has never been proven since technically you don't have a body anymore. Perhaps your ghost feels the heat. One can only hope now, with modern technology, that Purgatory is equipped with video games and laptops to help pass the time while you wait for the Heavenly gates to open. Coffee and tea would be nice too!)

At any rate, when my complaints about the heat became intolerable, and the air outside turned almost toxic, my parents would finally break down and put on the air-conditioner. I used to stand right in front of it and feel as though I had personally been delivered from the fires of Hell.

So, when it's really hot outside, don't kill yourself to try to exercise. One recent summer, the temperature was over one hundred degrees for almost an entire week. Needless to say, walking outside was out of the question, and so was going to the gym. No matter how many air-conditioners there were at the gym, they could never seem to keep up with the intense heat outside. I felt sure the earth's core had started to melt with that heat wave. One alternative is to go to an indoor mall and walk (but leave your credit card home so you won't be tempted to shop instead).

As I explained in the previous chapter, after years and years of searching, I did find the perfect gym for me—the Wellness Club at the local hospital. It's small, friendly and economical—just sixty-five dollars a month. (And still being quite the cheapskate, I try to go at least five times a week not only to feel great but to get my "money's worth." At five times a week, that's only three dollars and twenty-five cents every time I go!)

The secret is heading straight to the gym right after work. Do NOT go home first, because I guarantee you'll never go back out again. (I'm definitely not a morning person, so I would never try to get there before work.) It eventually becomes part of your routine and your car will automatically drive you there. Even if I've had a bad day at the office, I know that when I get to the Wellness Club, I'm going to see people I know and we can commiserate as we work out.

When I first joined, I started out with the treadmill—something nice and easy. After I felt comfortable with that, I graduated to the elliptical machine. It was really difficult at first and I found it extremely hard to do even ten minutes. But I stuck with it and would gradually increase the amount of time on that infernal machine. I now do up to thirty minutes, but anywhere from twenty to thirty minutes is a great workout.

I try to use the weight machines at least three times a week. Some days I can get through the circuit with no problem and other days, I'm struggling to finish. There's no rhyme or reason for this—some days are just better than others.

I would also recommend trying various exercise classes. My favorite class at the Wellness Club is Cardio Tone, which is a combination of some cardio and weight training. It's a small class and we have all become friends and actually go out to dinner occasionally. We're quite a diverse group as well—Christian, Jewish, and Muslim—and we all get along famously. It makes such a big difference when you know you're going to be working out with friends, and you can all moan and groan together for an hour.

Yoga is also a great way to stretch out the old body, and it's also strengthening and relaxing.

It's taken me nineteen years, but now I guess I am sort of a gym junkie. I try to go every day after work and sometimes on Saturdays. If I'm not at the gym, I'm walking outside or in the mall. I guess I've gotten to the point now that NOT working out seems very odd to me. Or it could be that my car is actually on automatic pilot—it just drives to the Wellness Club and I get out when it arrives there.

The bottom line is to not think about the fact that you have to do some type of activity. Just go and do it. The more you think about it, the more you might talk yourself out of it—the story of my life.

So besides the weather, the only other acceptable reasons to skip working out are sickness or a fancy event to attend. Otherwise, suck it up!

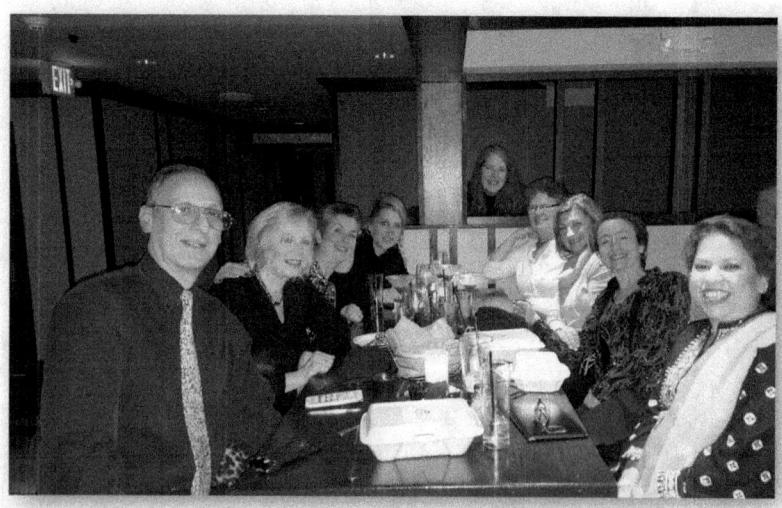

Our Cardio Tone Class enjoying dinner in Peekskill, NY, 2016
From left: Ed, Me, Kyle, Debbie (our instructor), Cynthia, Mary C., Joan, Leslie and Sabia

What Works for Me in Working in the Workouts

1. Most smart phones will track your steps for the day, or you can use a Fitbit or even a pedometer. Once you see how many (or how few) steps you're making, you'll want to challenge yourself and continually increase that number. If you do have a Fitbit, you'll get little rewards like the Boat Shoe or the Sneaker. Corny as it seems, getting those little rewards *is* a motivator.

2. At the beginning of each day, make it a point to do some type of activity. If you work full time, use part of your lunch hour to walk outside or at a nearby mall (but leave your credit card in your office so you won't be tempted to stop and shop). Take the stairs instead of the elevator, and make sure you get up and walk around the office every so often. (If you walk quickly, your boss will think you're in the middle of doing something really important.)

3. Go gym shopping. Most places will let you try it out for a week. Find one that's in your budget and that you like. Call your local hospital and ask if they have a gym or wellness club that is open to the public. Finding a place you like is half the battle.

4. Try to fit in strength training two or three times a week. You don't have to go to a gym for this—you can buy some free weights and do it at home. Strength training will tone your body and help with your metabolism.

5. Mix up your workouts. If you walk one day (treadmill or outside) do strength training the next day. Then maybe go back to walking or try the elliptical machine the following day. Bike riding outside is also a good option, as is inline skating. (I'm much too uncoordinated to try that, but it looks like fun.) An outdoor sport is another great option (but, again, I'm too much of a klutz for that).

6. Go dancing! Find bands or DJs that start early if you're an "old-timer" like me.

CHAPTER 5

Choosing Healthy Foods (Especially When Faced with Cheesecake)

by Mary T. Prenon

Oh Lord, Oh Lord, I am a sinner
I'll repent I promise, just after dinner.
I pray the greasy fat will die
Before it lands on my big thighs.
Amen.

So you're motivated and have hopefully found a gym or activity that you like. Now, let's talk about the healthy eating thing. I'm not going to sugarcoat this (no pun intended). Choosing healthy foods is damn hard work.

Let's face it—who in their right mind likes eating fruits and vegetables instead of fried chicken, French fries, pizza, egg rolls, cookies, cake, and candy bars? I don't care how good some people say they feel by eating healthy, because I know there's no one on this planet who can honestly tell me that a fruit cup is more delicious than a fresh, creamy, exquisite piece of New York–style cheesecake. Fattening food is scrumptious, and there's no way in hell that low-fat food will ever be able to compete. It's that simple.

Unfortunately, we're screwed if we eat too much fattening food. High-fat foods have been linked to diabetes, heart disease, cancer, etc., so unless you want to check out of life early, you have to eat healthy. And, after a while, the healthy food will actually taste really good. (Still not as good as cheesecake, though).

The big problem with trying to eat healthy is that all too often our stomachs tell our brains what to do. So, how do we make our brains the boss? That's a question I still struggle with every day of my life, but over the years, I have learned a couple of things. One is to keep the stomach happy by not letting it run on empty. When the stomach is empty, it rules the body and makes you do the craziest things.

Too many times, I have been guilty of not properly filling up the tank in the morning so I won't crave the wrong things the rest of the day. Filling up the tank on weekday mornings can be really difficult if, like me, you're constantly running out the door at the last minute to get to the office on time.

As I explained before, in my "radio days" I would never eat breakfast since I had to be at work by 5:00 a.m. for the morning shift. We would make our local police calls before the 6:00 a.m. news to see if anything dramatic happened overnight. Then we'd type up our newscasts using actual typewriters! (Yes, it was the eighties and there were very few computers.) We were so busy that we rarely ate anything before 9:00 a.m. when morning drive was over. At that point, anything was consumed. Besides the leftover bagels from the sales department's meetings, there was always abundant free food at press conferences. The reporters would usually gather at the food table and inhale volumes of edibles both before and after the press conference.

As I said, this "radio mentality" is still with me today. There's just something about free stuff that makes us want to devour it just because it is free.

Years after, when I was working at the ad agency, stress and the lack of adequate hours in the day often led to unhealthy eating habits. One day in particular, I really went into an eating frenzy. It started with oversleeping then dragging my gargantuan butt into the office to make final preparations for a morning meeting with a client. Confident the client would serve some semblance of breakfast, I left the office with an empty stomach. Upon arrival at the meeting, I was horrified to see an empty conference room table. Not even a breadcrumb. "My God," I thought. "How the hell am I supposed to think about writing their ads if they're not going to feed me?"

But wait—it got worse. After that meeting, I had a noon meeting with another client. Surely, this one would have some morsels of sustenance to offer me. The good news was, there was food. The bad news—it was doughnuts. Out of the corner of my eye, I spied a doughnut with pink icing. At first, I tried to ignore it, but the hour was late, and I still had not had my breakfast. I fought the urge to eat the donut, dutifully concentrating on the annual report I was to write. But, alas, my concentration was broken by my stomach crying out in pain, "Feed me, feed me, you fool! I can't go on! I'm dying!" With that, the pink circle of life was thrust into my pie hole.

If you can believe this, the day got even worse. After the meeting, the client offered me some candy that she kept in a large bowl on her desk. She said she hardly ever ate it. Well, that was obvious as she was a very thin woman. How the hell could she keep a huge bowl of candy on her desk and not eat it? I simply failed to comprehend. My face would have been buried in that bowl and wouldn't come up for air until every last morsel had been consumed. God, even the thought of it was exciting. Alas, I indulged in the candy and by the end of the day, I felt extremely nauseous. I vowed *never again* to be a piggy. Needless to say, that didn't last long.

Holidays are the most difficult time to make healthy eating choices. The over-indulgence begins with Thanksgiving and ends about a week after New Year's...with an additional ten pounds. Easter is no better. I have failed the "chocolate rabbit" test many times.

Once I took a healthy cooking class in another relentless effort to turn my life around. While the food we cooked was healthy, it was also practically inedible. Grilled tofu and a bean salad are not my idea of a dinner. Hell, if this is what's considered healthy, let me eat junk and die happy. In fact, the food was so disgusting that I was forced to seek solace in a bucket of fried chicken later that night.

Sometimes you might think you're eating healthy, but actually you're not. Take a close look at food labels. Look at the amount of sugars, sodium, and carbohydrates. Try to stick with foods that are low in sugar (less than 10 mg), carbs (less than 25 mg), and sodium (less than 400 mg). Excess sodium can cause high blood pressure, which is no good for the old "ticker." Too much sugar can spike your triglycerides, which could lead to high cholesterol. It could also be a factor for diabetes. (The American Heart Association recommends no more than 2,300 milligrams of sodium a day, with about 1,500 as the ideal amount.)

It took me years—almost twenty of them—to finally get the whole "healthy eating" thing. My weekends were typically pizza on Friday night, Chinese on Saturday night and maybe a cooked meal on Sundays. Eating out at restaurants too much is also a good way to add more calories, salt, carbs and sugar. The breadbasket alone can be a killer.

One thing that has really helped me is a free app called "My Fitness Pal." It asks for your current weight and how much you want to lose. Then it sets up a daily guide for the amount of sugar, protein, carbs, fat, sodium, etc., you need. It'll let you know when you're getting close to your goals, and, of course, it will definitely let you know when you're over. I tend to eat a lot of fruit, so I usually go over my sugar limits a little. However, I figure fruit is way better than cheesecake.

The other great—or maybe not so great—thing about My Fitness Pal is that it will tell you what you may not want to know. Lots of times, food that you think is healthy is actually anything BUT healthy. You may think a veggie sandwich from a popular chain eatery would be a perfect lunch, but after looking it up on My Fitness Pal, and the restaurant's website, you find that it has over 1,000 milligrams of sodium and more than sixty carbs! Yikes!

Yes, it can be a pain to look up foods, but in reality, it takes just seconds and it's well worth the time. However when I'm having one of those "I'm famished" days, I often fear that My Fitness Pal will suddenly grow arms and start slapping me if I shove breads or sweets into my mouth.

I'm not a nutritionist, so you may want to consult one to help you on your journey. But be careful. I have met with some nutritionists before—some had great advice while others didn't. Some actually advocated eating lots of cereals and breads, and some put too little emphasis on exercising.

I like to seek out various opinions, so I read everything I can about healthy eating. Here's what I've learned in a nutshell: fruits, veggies, whole grains, beans, nuts seeds, lean meats, and fish—good. Processed or fried foods, white breads and pastas, fatty and salty foods, lots of red meat, abundant sweets—bad. The jury is still out on dairy—some say eat it, others say don't. Here's my take—I stick to low-sugar Greek yogurt and skim milk. I do like cheese, but I eat it sparingly. And yes, I most certainly DO imbibe frozen yogurt. I know it's high in sugar, but it's my weekend treat. Unfortunately, I can't do ice cream anymore. Once my gall bladder was removed, ice cream plays havoc with my intestines. The last few times I ate ice cream I spent the rest of the evening in the bathroom. Enough said!

OK, so let's start with breakfast. As Mom always said, breakfast is the most important meal of the day. It fills up your tank, and starts to fuel you for the day. For breakfast, stay away from anything sugary like some cereals, pastries, bagels, etc., and stick with a low-carb, low-sugar Greek yogurt or oatmeal, fruit, eggs, whole grain breads or English muffins with peanut butter for protein.

When it comes to lunch, I have become the "salad queen" at the office. Because buying lunch can get very expensive, I usually bring a bagged salad and throw some grilled chicken or shrimp on top. I've also taken a liking to snap peas with a little hummus. Low-sodium soup is great in the colder months—check the organic aisle of your local supermarket. Sometimes, I break down and buy a sandwich—usually on Fridays—as my reward for eating salads all week. I try to stick with whole grain breads, though.

For snacks, I have become addicted to apple slices with peanut butter and some low sodium popcorn. You can also choose veggies like carrots, celery, or peppers with hummus.

For dinner, I opt for chicken, turkey, or fish with two helpings of veggies. Sometimes, I'll make brown rice or sweet potatoes. Full disclosure—I am *not* a person who weighs my food. I recently had a discussion with Dr. K about this and just told him flat out—that's not how I roll. Here's the deal—I work like a dog all day in the office. Then I work out like an even bigger dog at the gym for an hour every night. I'm not coming home exhausted, and then throwing a piece of chicken on a scale. Sorry, not happening. I always buy medium-sized chicken breasts or a medium-sized piece of fish. With all of the calories I burn at the gym, it's not going to kill me to eat a whole piece of protein. Maybe I'm wrong, but I have lost almost fifty pounds this way. (Of course, that's after wasting about seventeen years being lazy and eating all the wrong crap!)

When I do have events to attend, I can now completely avoid the free food, since most of it is fried, fatty and loaded with salt. I make sure I have a healthy snack like nuts or some veggies and hummus before I attend these events so I won't be tempted to indulge. Also, having AFib is always a good built-in reminder that eating the "sodium bombs" will have the old ticker doing the Mambo all night. I also remind myself that while I'm far from being rich, I'm financially comfortable enough to buy food and don't need to rely on free stuff. (Unless, of course, they're giving away a smart TV or some other electronic wonder. Then I'll be running for the free stuff.)

I've also finally learned to take it easy with the sweets. If someone brings cookies to the office, I'll have no more than two. After years and years of eating badly, I now realize that sweets are my addiction and it will only lead to a downward spiral. At my age, too much sugar can make my heart race. So when it comes to sodium and sugar, I'm basically screwed!

Even if you don't have AFib now, it could be lurking right around the corner. It can affect any age, sex, or race, so no one is immune. Like I've said before, fear is always a good motivator to avoid unhealthy foods. And you can still have a great time at an event without relying on the food. Don't make that your sole purpose for attending. Challenge yourself to mingle and meet as many new people as possible. It can help your social life and your career at the same time. After a while, you won't even miss the food. I know, I can't believe I just said that. (Again, it took me nineteen years to figure that out!)

I also travel quite a bit—up to Cape Cod, Massachusetts and down to Pennsylvania. Making healthy food choices on the road is even harder because all the rest stops are filled with junk. When traveling to the Cape, I always stop at Fresh City on the Massachusetts Turnpike. They have salads and wraps, so you can get a much better selection of healthy foods. It's funny though. Every time I'm there, the line for McDonald's is extremely long, while there's practically no line for Fresh City. I guess people are so familiar with McDonald's that they know what they're going to get and many, I guess, are just too skeptical to make a change and try something new.

If the only thing you can find is fast food, try to choose a salad selection. Most places post the calories, fat, salt, etc., so you can actually see what you're eating (that is, if you really want to!). What I found interesting is that recently when I was at a rest stop, there was a store offering "healthy" sandwiches. However, when I looked at the sodium content, it was about 1,100 milligrams for one sandwich! Not so healthy. I ended up getting a grilled chicken sandwich from a fast-food place, only to discover afterward that the hamburger probably would have been a better choice. It actually had way less sodium than the chicken sandwich.

If you're looking for a snack, I'd go with unsalted nuts, or a low-sugar/low-sodium protein bar. Fruit is another good choice. Of course, you can always bring an apple or some other fruit with you.

I actually eat the healthiest when I'm at Cape Cod. Because of all the fresh fish, my diet is basically some type of fish every night. (Of course, I do love my frozen yogurt, too!) My cousins Ave and Mary live there, as does my friend Doreen. Yes, we all do enjoy our "eating fests" there, but there's also so much activity, like swimming, hiking, biking and of course, dancing!

So what's the bottom line—do I eat healthy every single day? No. Do I screw up a lot? Yes. Are these lifestyle changes always going to suck? No. Believe it or not, once you get your body used to eating healthy, it will start to crave the healthy foods. I know it sounds bizarre, but it's true. Your body is pretty smart—if you treat it right, it will let you know what it needs.

Every day is still a huge struggle for me. I don't know whether it's because of the bloodline of alcoholics in our family, but I have to tell you the sugar cravings are so bad sometimes that I just want to scream. I remember years ago comparing stories about addictions with my cousin Charlie, who passed several years ago from a heart condition. We were very close—he was like a brother to me. We used to fight when we were little, but when we got older, we would hang out together, going to concerts and attending the same junior college.

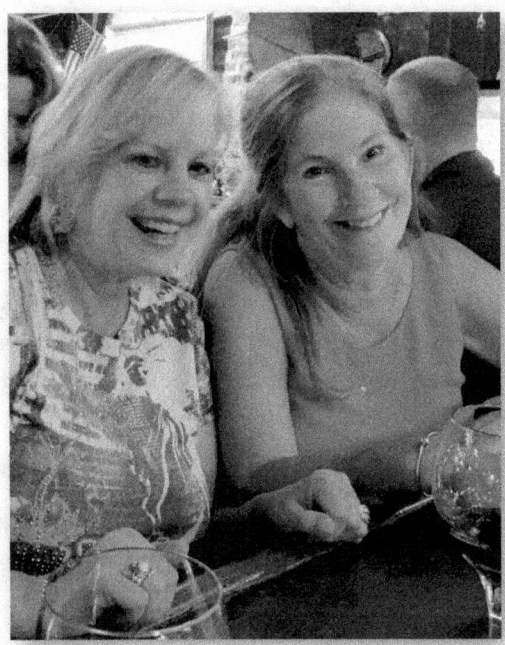

From left, Me and Doreen having cocktails in Cape Cod, MA, 2017

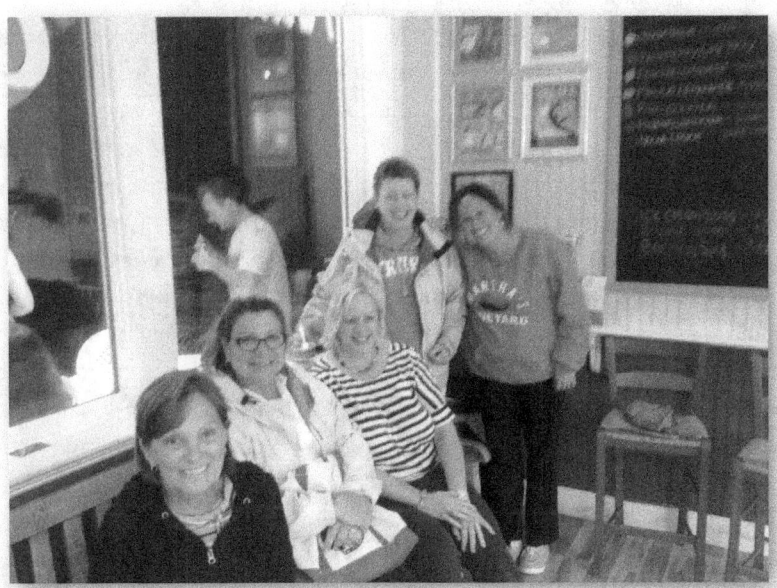

From left, Cousin Pat, Cousin Mary, Me, Cousin Ave and Cousin Leanne
at an ice cream/frozen yogurt shop in Cape Cod, MA, 2014

When he went off to join the armed services, we used to write crazy, funny letters to each other. (Again, before day days of email).

Charlie lived in California for many years and our letter writing continued. Unfortunately, he got heavily involved with alcohol and drugs and was even homeless for a while. He used to fascinate me with stories about his life in a "tent city." Finally, he moved back east and started to get his life together.

As a recovering alcoholic, Charlie battled with drinking just as much as I battled with eating. One day we were talking about the fact that many times when I went out to a bar or club, I wouldn't have an alcoholic drink. He looked at me completely puzzled and said, "How can you go to a bar and not drink?" To which I replied, "How can you go to a bakery and not eat?" It was a moment of enlightenment as we now fully understood each other's addictions.

(There's a quick side story about Charlie that I must include here because he definitely would have wanted me to do that. Besides his alcohol addiction, Charlie struggled with his sexual identity for many years. Finally, he felt comfortable enough to legally change his name to Carla, and began gearing up for the transition process. At any rate, Carla and I would often go out to drag shows in Rehoboth Beach, Delaware, where he lived. One night when we were watching the show, a rather drunken woman came up to me and began looking me up and down. I started to feel uncomfortable and politely told her that I was straight. She said nothing, but left. OK, I thought, no harm done. As I turned around, I saw Carla and his "girls" laughing hysterically. When I asked him what was so funny, he said they had told the drunk woman that I "transitioned" a year ago! "You told her I used to be a man?" I screamed. They just kept laughing! Well, I suppose I should be flattered since the woman obviously thought the surgeon had done an outstanding job turning me into a woman! You iust gotta love Charlie/Carla and I really do miss him/her and his/her practical jokes.)

OK, back to reality now. There are still many times I really do miss the foods I used to eat, and I fantasize about having my old life back. I actually have colorful dreams about pies—rows and rows of different kinds like Boston cream, cherry, apple, and blueberry!

However, the reality is if I was miraculously presented with a pizza, Buffalo wings, fried chicken, Chinese food, and a cheesecake, I would have to turn them away because I know they'd be toxic to my system now. (Well, OK, just a tiny piece of cheesecake!)

So how do you get to this point? Well, I may not the best person to ask since it took me almost two decades to say "no" to the crappy food. But here's my simple suggestion—start out by focusing on any type of exercise like walking, biking, or even housework (God forbid). Believe me, you will begin to feel good—tired, but good—and then you'll be much less likely to ruin all the hard work you accomplished by eating unhealthy foods.

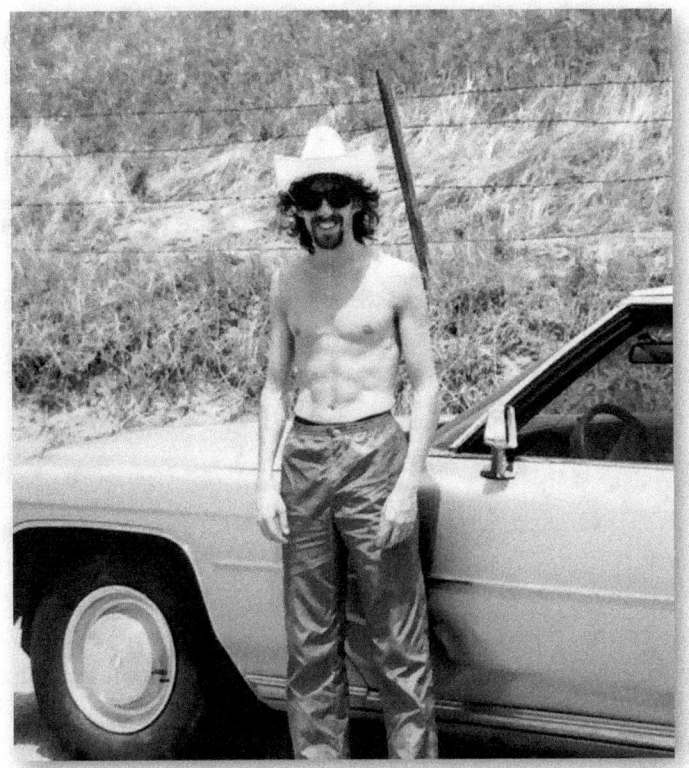

My cousin Charlie in San Jose, CA, 1987

Of course, this could backfire like it did for me so many, many times. In the past, I'd work out and then use that as justification for eating junk. "Hey, I just burned off a lot of calories, so I can reward myself." Ah, NO! The fact I failed to realize is that I was completely screwing myself over by putting back all of the calories I just worked off. I would get really pissed off and then depressed.

The trick is to get a good workout in and then really think about what you're going to eat later. Plan it out, and prepare the healthy meal. Full disclosure—you may not like this in the beginning. In fact you may hate it and be particularly grumpy for the rest of the day—or week. But stick with it. Get in a couple more walks or gym workouts during the week and it will start to change the way you feel about yourself. Then the light in your head will turn on and you'll suddenly find yourself walking toward the salad bar. Every day may not be like this, but you'll soon notice that the more days you exercise, the more times you'll choose to eat healthy meals.

It's not rocket science—it's actually pretty simple. That's why it's so important to make regular exercise a habit. It's the key to turning around your whole attitude toward food.

At the end of this book, you'll find my humble suggestions for what to eat for breakfast, lunch, dinner, and snacks. Next, what happens when you do screw up—that is, the story of my life!

What Works for Me in Making Healthy Eating Choices

1. Start out with a healthy breakfast. If you start the day out right, you'll tend to stay on the right path the rest of your day. (Of course, if someone brings brownies to the office, you're totally screwed.) If you do eat unhealthy goodies, it's not the end of the world. Do some walking at lunch and eat healthy for the rest of the day. One wrong move in the morning doesn't have to mess up the whole day.

2. Don't let yourself get too hungry. Make sure you have some healthy snacks like nuts or fruit between breakfast and lunch, and then again between lunch and dinner.

3. Drink plenty of water. I drink an average of eight to twelve glasses a day. You'll go to the bathroom more often, but drinking water fills you up, keeps you hydrated, and makes your skin look great. It's also a great way of helping to prevent AFib.

4. Keep track of what you're eating. It can be a pain, but you'll get used to it. You can download free apps like My Fitness Pal to see the calories, sugar, salt, carbs, fat, etc., that you're eating. This can really help to keep you on track.

5. If you're like me and you have an occasional bout of AFib, that's a built-in reminder to watch your sodium intake. The American Heart Association recommends consuming no more than 1,500 milligrams of sodium a day. Adopting a low-sodium diet really helped me shed the tonnage.

CHAPTER 6
Dealing with Setbacks

This is the longest chapter of the book because I have lived through almost twenty years of setbacks. I still have setbacks today, but I've finally learned to manage them better. "Setback" is my middle name. If I had a dime for every setback I've had, I'd be a billionaire. Someone once told me that a setback is a setup for a comeback, and I think there's some truth to that.

Why do we have setbacks? The answer is easy—they're part of life. Sometimes you can eat all the right foods and get in your exercise, and then something blows it all to hell. It can be anything—a bad day at work, a disagreement with someone, money troubles, a breakup, or just getting sick and tired of not being able to eat what you want.

For me, holidays are setbacks. Take Halloween, for instance. I wait until the last minute to buy the candy so it won't be around for me to eat. I also try to buy candy I hate so I'll be less tempted. The problem is, there's not much out there that I hate.

My downfall is candy corn. Candy corn is like my own personal crack. I've always loved it, and it seems every year I buy it and eat it until I'm sick. Then I vow never to eat it again (until next Halloween). The only good thing about overeating Halloween candy is that the candies nowadays are bite sized.

When I was a kid, people gave out the big "nickel" candy bars, which today probably cost about two dollars (if you live in New York). I would go out trick-or-treating at about six o'clock at night, come home at seven thirty to unload the first bagful of goodies, and then go out again for a second batch. Back then I never gained weight, but practically every tooth in my mouth had a filling.

Then there's Thanksgiving and the prequel to the Holidays. The office can be a cauldron of setbacks with daily delicacies delivered from clients and, of course, the

Holiday luncheon. The luncheon was the king of all setbacks. In fact, one year was so bad I wrote a poem about it.

Tons of Love This Holiday Season
by Mary T. Prenon

We had our Christmas lunch today and now I'm really huge.
I split my pants. I broke my bra. I can't fit in my shoes.

I sat down at the table, and I tied the feedbag on
Through salad, soup, and entree, plus coffee and bonbon.

I waddled from the table like a hippo on the move.
I came back to the office just to eat some more junk food.

And now I'm near exhaustion, and my jaws are feeling limp.
I really wish I hadn't had that extra piece of shrimp.

So farewell friends, it's time to go, my taxi ride is here—
A big, bright yellow forklift from the people at John Deere.

Christmas and the Holidays are the worst time for setbacks. Not only do they confront you with a myriad of delectable, sugary delights, but there's the added stress of dealing with your family. Dad and I often got into nasty fights about my eating too much and his drinking too much. We eventually agreed that both subjects were taboo.

Speaking of Dad, there's no greater setback than when you lose a loved one. Dad had never really been sick his whole life, but in the end, the smoking and drinking took their toll, even though he had stopped drinking for about seven years prior to his passing.

I was forty-two in the spring of 1999 when he was rushed to the hospital for a burst appendix. Later we learned that the appendix was cancerous and that he also had a small brain tumor. Added to this were his failing lungs and liver, plus a heart attack. Dad died on May 22 of that year from his many health complications.

Although my family was prepared, we still took it pretty hard. To this day, I still can't believe he's gone. Dad was always healthy, and he was so sharp-witted and had a great sense of humor, even in his hospital bed. I'm amazed that he made it to eighty years old, though. He drank, smoked, never exercised, and never ate the right foods. I guess he had good genes.

After his funeral in suburban Philadelphia, the reality of what had happened hit me hard. I was alone now. Mom had passed in 1993 of a heart attack, and I had no sisters, no brothers, no husband, and no kids. Talk about a setback!

Dad and I had become a lot closer since Mom died, but I wouldn't call our family close-knit by any stretch. I had a lot of issues with my father. His drinking almost drove us completely apart, but I can look back now and admire him for having the courage to quit cold turkey and stay clean for seven years. How did he do it? I often wish I had the same strength he had when it came to my own addiction to sweets.

When I returned to New York, I made a decision to get myself back on track, physically and mentally. To be mentally strong, I would have to become physically strong as well, since body and mind are designed to work together (or so I've heard).

Things were going great for a while, and then BLAM!—summer arrived. As I mentioned earlier, I am not a fan of hot weather. The older I get, the more the heat bothers me. Many of my friends and colleagues talk about retiring to North Carolina, Florida, or Arizona. I will retire in Alaska, Nova Scotia, or Iceland.

In addition to hot weather being a setback to exercising outdoors or indoors (sometimes the air-conditioners in the gym just can't keep the place cool enough), summer is also a time for great church carnivals filled with delicacies like meatball wedges, Italian ices, soft pretzels, zeppoles, and, of course, funnel cakes. It's a time when I squeeze into my elastic-waist shorts and tie on a feedbag.

My summer overeating binges would often lead right into Halloween, Thanksgiving, and Christmas overeating binges. Dad's death made 1999 a particularly bad year for me in this regard, but it did spur me to write another poem.

Another Year Shot to Hell
by Mary T. Prenon

The millennium has come and gone, and I'm still fat and broke.
I'm overweight. I got no cash. My life's a freaking joke.

The year 2000 was to be the start of my new life.
With working out and eating right, eliminating strife.

Now this year's shot, and nothing's changed. I'm right back at the start.
My weight is up, the market's down, my budget's off the charts.

No fancy home, no skimpy clothes, no weekends at the beach.
When I look into the mirror now, I simply want to screech!

So here's to failure and fiasco in the millennium.
Let's toast to being rich and thin for year 2001.

Sometimes setbacks come in the guise of comfort, especially after an embarrassing moment. When I was with the ad agency, one of our clients was a large museum, and I had an appointment to meet the new director. I was dressed in a new dapper pantsuit and new shoes, with makeup on, and I was having a good hair day. Unfortunately, my new shoes didn't quite hit it off with the polished floors outside the director's office and (how predictable) BOOM!—down I went as the director and a cadre of people looked on. Hey, can I make an appearance or what? Obviously, one can clearly see the need to indulge in an all-you-can-eat Chinese buffet after such a catastrophe. (A quick observation about all-you-can-eat Chinese buffets—did you ever notice that most of the customers are "nutritionally challenged," while the entire wait staff is thin?)

I once attended a birthday party at a Chinese buffet. Not wanting to be rude, I filled up my plate again and again. I'm talking chicken wings, spare ribs, egg rolls—the whole nine yards. I did eat healthy—chicken and broccoli. By the end of the night, I was ready to call the local forklift company to take me home. Just as I was approaching the door to leave, I felt something snap, and my left boob headed south. My bra broke! I'm not kidding. The plastic piece on the strap that holds you in place snapped. Talk about being lopsided! Fortunately, I was on my way out and managed to get to the car before completely drooping.

Another fun and exciting event that turned into a setback was the grand opening of a new health club for one of our clients at the advertising agency. I distinctly remember they served marble cheesecake. I guess the psychology behind that was to get everyone fat so they'd join. The club was beautiful except for all the mirrors. I couldn't get away from myself and that big butt following me around all night. There was one woman there with a perfect body, parading around in a short black skirt with slits. I'm sure every woman in the place hated her. "Why can't I have the kind of body that women hate?" I thought. Instead, I realized I had the kind of body that men hate.

Setbacks aren't always caused by overeating at a restaurant or a party. Sometimes even going to the doctor's office can trigger a setback. At one of my annual ob-gyn checkups, I was required to do the unthinkable—step onto a scale. It had been more than a year since I had completed such a horrific task, but at the insistence of the nurse, I sheepishly crept onto that infernal gadget, hoping…uh, make that praying… that the number wouldn't embarrass me. Wrong! (My philosophy has always been don't let the scale rule your life—it's more about how you feel, how you look, and how you fit into your clothes that counts. Unfortunately, the nurse wasn't buying this argument.) When I finally got the courage to look, the number I saw—198—sent me into a two-day meltdown. It couldn't be true. The scale must be wrong. It was telling me that I was two pounds shy of 200? While 200 is not so terrible in the grand scheme of things—it's a hell of a lot better than 300 or 400—it was still forty extra pounds hanging around my butt, boobs, stomach, and thighs. (Note: This was not the highest the scale ever climbed. I know I had gained much more over the years, but I was never able to confirm my top number due to my refusal to step on the scale for years at a time.)

Fortunately, my meltdown occurred over the weekend, so it didn't cost me any time from work. I basically spent that Saturday and Sunday bawling my eyes out, looking at myself in the mirror in utter disgust, and eating very little of anything (which is really stupid, because that only slowed down my metabolism, making weight loss even more difficult). Eventually, the reality of life—nations at war, children in need, cancer, etc.—took over, and I came to my senses. I realized that my problems are nothing compared to what some people are dealing with. I was alive and relatively healthy— just a little overweight.

The meltdown came and went, and I became more determined than ever to eat healthy, exercise, and get back into shape. But, of course, life has a way of changing your plans. As I was hanging my new fall curtains one Sunday afternoon, I stupidly decided to stand on the back of the sofa instead of moving the sofa out of the way and standing on a steady chair. Well, you can guess the rest of the story. Yep, my foot slipped as I was stepping down onto the sofa cushion, my body went into a curious array of convulsions, and I hit the back of my head on the coffee table and landed smack on the floor with a loud thud. My neighbors next door probably thought there was an earthquake, or that someone had dropped an A-bomb.

At first, I couldn't move my left foot at all—shards of pain shot out in every direction. Meantime, my right wrist sported a nice, juicy bump. After about five minutes, I managed to get up and hobble into the kitchen to make ice bags for my hand and foot. A few hours later, I was at the hospital emergency room, being treated for fractures. Exercising, even walking, was out for at least a month.

Following this bone-breaking episode, my luck managed to get even worse. It's almost like a black cloud was following me around. Since I was now "booted," i.e., equipped with a "Herman Munster"–style shoe, I tried to limit my walking as much as possible. Unfortunately, this meant using a valet to park my car when meeting with some of my clients. I never liked valet parking, and I'll give you one guess for what's coming next. Bingo! The valet crashed my car. Yep—I was on a real lucky streak. The good news was that no one got hurt. The bad news was a $5,000-plus repair job for my car. After having another mini-nervous breakdown, I was elated to discover that the valet company would pay for the damage, as well as reimburse me for the towing and rental car.

But wait—there's more. I couldn't work out, my car was in the shop, the fat was growing, and then I got my very first toothache. It was a beauty. The dull, throbbing pain required an immediate trip to the dentist and a subsequent root canal. While the pain to my tooth was almost unbearable, the pain to my wallet was even worse.

Eventually, I recovered from the fractures and the toothache, and I managed to pick myself up and get back in the game of healthy living again—until the next setback, of course.

This time it came in the form of a gala to end all galas. A major real estate developer came to suburban New York City for the grand opening of a disgustingly expensive new high-rise condo building. It was the kind of building that's completely out of reach for commoners like me.

The ad agency I worked for handled the publicity for this ostentatious display of wealth, and the event was also a fundraiser for a local hospital. I had the best seat in the house for most of the night. I was stationed outside at the press table, checking everyone in and biting my nails in the hopes that all the press I invited would show up.

Public relations is such a stressful job. If a ton of media show up at an event, you're a queen. If they don't, you're a hideous, evil troll. What a crappy way to earn a living. Well, it could have been worse. I could have been cleaning the elephant cages at the zoo.

Following the check-ins, I made my way into the building for the program. The speeches (and a lot of pontificating) went on for almost an hour as my stomach groaned with hunger. Finally, the bullshit stopped, and we could eat. A stampede to the food stations ensued. It wasn't pretty, but eat I did, and I completely blew my healthy eating plan. Hell, I was starving. I tried to control myself with the desserts and ate half of only two small portions.

After that ordeal, I continued to remain in the "fat lane," but I hoped the thought of walking down the aisle again would catapult me out of it. No, not as a bride—God forbid—but as a bridesmaid. My boyfriend Tom's brother, Paul, and his fiancée, Gina, were getting married, and I was asked to be a bridesmaid. I graciously accepted, despite the fact that I'd probably be the world's oldest bridesmaid.

Gina and I went shopping for bridesmaid's dresses, and she chose a beautiful maroon dress. When I just about fit into a size sixteen, the bridal consultant suggested a size eighteen, which I adamantly refused. "No," I said. "Absolutely not. I will lose enough weight in time and fit into this just fine. In fact, I may even need to get a smaller size by then." (Pause here for laughter.)

A few months later I picked up the dress, confident that I would be swimming in it. Much to my horror, it was still quite tight. Desperate for help, I rushed the dress to a tailor, begging to have the sides let out just a pinch. When I went to pick up the dress from the tailor the morning of the wedding, she told me she had forgotten to do it, and asked me to come back in an hour. I was a little freaked out, but I agreed and ran some errands. I returned home to discover that the tailor had left two frantic phone messages saying there wasn't any material to let out and that the dress could not be altered. What?! Apparently, there was extra material on the inside seams near the bottom of the dress, but not at the top. I officially went into panic mode.

I picked up the dress, saving sixty-five dollars on the alterations, and did the only thing I could do—pray. Fortunately, someone was listening. I skipped the bra and furiously held my breath and sucked in my gut while Tom's mother, Joanne, painstakingly zipped me from the back and Tom stood in front of me, shoving my boobs into the dress. It was a truly hilarious moment, even though I felt like crying.

But what really saved me was the matching shawl that I had purchased a week earlier. That was the best twenty-dollar investment I'd ever made in my life. It covered up the overflow of boob and subsequent arm fat caused by the pushing and scrunching.

After wearing the dress for a while, I found I could breathe normally again—that was, until I started to eat. At that point, I felt the dress tightening around my upper torso and wondered if this was the same sensation one would feel being squeezed to death by a giant python. I wondered if it would cut off blood circulation and make my entire upper body turn blue. I wondered if anyone else in the room was as uncomfortable as I was. By 10:00 p.m., I couldn't take it anymore and changed into a regular dress I had brought with me in case the bridesmaid's dress became unbearable. Let's face it, my bridesmaid days were over.

Again, I managed to get back in the game for a while—exercising and trying to eat healthy foods, but unfortunately, I had yet another setback. My ad agency colleagues and I were on our way to a client meeting (which happened to be a hospital) when I had my first-ever panic attack—and it was a whopper!

The weather had been very warm, so I wasn't concerned when my hot flashes kicked in. But when I couldn't catch my breath, I got a bit concerned. I felt trapped— like I had to get out of the car—and I had a mild session of crying and heavy breathing. I was experiencing my first panic attack. Fortunately, I was able to snap out of it by relying on yoga breaths, and I was in decent shape by the time we got to the hospital. My boss, on the other hand, was completely freaked out by it.

It's funny how things happen for a reason. That crazy incident was actually my wake-up call to find a career that was less stressful—and less damaging to my health. Starting a new career at the age of forty-eight definitely constitutes a setback. One of my clients at the ad agency was a fabulous new spa in the Berkshires in western Massachusetts, and I was up there quite a bit to set up press interviews. I fully admit that I am a "spa junkie" and loved being in the spa atmosphere. "What a peaceful place to work," I thought. And that's when it hit me—I would give up my crazy ad agency job for a more serene work experience.

I gave my notice, cashed in some CDs, and enrolled in a six-month esthetician course at a local spa school. Many people told me I was brave to do that, but I believe some of them secretly thought I was more crazy than brave. Either way, it turned out to be one of the best decisions of my life. And, yes, it did result in some setbacks for healthy living.

One day after school I decided to visit a friend with a one-year-old baby. While I do like babies, they never seem to like me—they cry and scream every time I hold them. That's why I try to avoid holding them at all costs. Well, my friend and I were sitting and talking when she suddenly felt sick and had to run outside to hurl. I was left holding the baby and, yes, scream she did.

I spent the next half hour running outside to check on my friend then back inside to try to comfort the crying baby, who I had placed in a playpen. I must have looked like an idiot, picking up every toy in sight and violently shaking it in hopes of calming the little tyke. When something finally worked, I'd run outside again, only to hear the caterwauling from the playpen once again. At one point, I picked the baby up, and she actually remained quiet for at least a minute before exercising her rather vibrant vocal chords. (Maybe it was because I held her like I hold my cats. You can see where this is going.) Long story short—mom and baby were both OK. As for me, it ended with an emergency stop at Burger King.

Sometimes, thinking about where you are in your life can be a setback. I'm divorced, I have no children and no brothers and sisters, and my parents have passed. If I sit around and obsess about that, I will be depressed, and the last thing I'll want to do is eat healthy and exercise.

While I am a "mom" to my cat Oliver, I often wonder what my life would be like if I were "on the other side," i.e., married with children. (And, of course, I know there are many married moms out there wondering what life would be like sans husband and children.) Sometimes when I'm at the mall, I'll see a seemingly happy family walking by smiling and laughing. But just when I start to think, "Yes, maybe I'd enjoy that," the crying and screaming erupts in the distance as the parents and kids obviously have a disagreement over a toy, candy, or the fact that the kids have had enough shopping for the day. It's then that I realize my life is right where it's supposed to be. Sure, the cats will whine sometimes, but I don't have to worry about dragging them to the mall, checking their homework, and being sure to put boots and gloves on their paws.

One drawback to having animals instead of children is that kids will eventually grow out of wearing diapers, graduate from college, and move out. Cats will never grow out of using the litter box and never move out. If you have a cat or dog, you'll be shoveling crap for the rest of their lives.

I have never been very "motherly" except when it comes to taking care of my cats. Is that normal? I guess it's normal for me. Having children is a huge responsibility, and people shouldn't have them just because it's something they're "supposed to do." It should be something they want to do and a responsibility they're ready and willing to take on. Does the fact that I didn't want this responsibility make me selfish? Sometimes I think it does. But then I think it would have been worse for me to do something just because society expected it from me. That may be one reason so many marriages break up and so many kids have problems.

In January 2007, at age forty-nine, just when I thought things were going to settle down, I faced another terrible setback—the loss of my godmother, my dear Aunt "Tiny," due to a major stroke. Aunt Tiny, whose real name is Catherine, was given her nickname when she was a child. The name stuck because, in fact, she was quite tiny.

Aunt Tiny would often drop subtle hints to me about eating too much, which for her meant two raisins instead of one. But despite her petite stature, Tiny was no pushover and usually got in the last word at family arguments. In a lot of ways, she was a woman before her time, having chosen a career over marriage and children. She even once worked for the Pinkerton Detective Agency, then for Amtrak. She told me the money was good, but I had to go and be a poor journalist instead.

Tiny loved to travel. She went all over the United States and Europe, and she always brought home lots of souvenirs. Of course, many of those trips were to religious places. She was a devout Catholic, but she also loved to have fun. She smoked and had many a "highball" cocktail. She had a dry sense of humor and came out with some real memorable one-liners.

We were always close, but when Mom passed away in 1993, Aunt Tiny became even more important to me. She would come up to New York to see me, and we'd go to shows and out to dinner and enjoy our cocktails. We had our fights, too. She used to tell me I was getting too fat, but anyone looked fat next to Aunt Tiny. She weighed a little over one hundred pounds.

We once had a big fight about my weight. We were at my cousin's wedding, and after one too many cocktails, Aunt Tiny went around telling everyone in the family exactly what she thought about them. I was deemed "too fat" (as were the majority of the wedding attendees), a cousin's hair was insulted, and it went downhill from there. I was so angry with her I didn't speak to her for a week. She finally wrote me a letter of apology. At the end of the letter she said she would always love me—even if I was fat. You gotta love that!

Aunt Tiny was eighty-four when she passed. It was fortunate that she went quickly. She was a very smart cookie, and living with the effects of a large stroke like the one she had would have destroyed her, even though she was never one to get stressed out. As long as she had a cup of coffee, a doughnut, and her crossword puzzle, she was in Heaven. In fact, she's probably enjoying those three things in Heaven right now. Viva, Aunt Tiny!

My point is that personal loss affects us in different ways. Many people can't eat, while others turn to food for comfort. I was one of the latter people. I managed to pack on the pounds again, even though I could still hear Aunt Tiny saying, "You're getting too fat!"

A few months after Aunt Tiny passed, my beloved cat Justin was diagnosed with cancer. He was only eight years old, so I decided to try chemotherapy. It didn't work, and he became so weak I had to put him down. It was an awful time for me, and, of course, being healthy was the last thing on my mind. In July of that year, I adopted a kitten, Melody, who became the annoying little sister to my other cat, Muffin.

Later that year, the thing that got me started back on the right road again was planning for my fiftieth birthday. My closest lifelong friends and I were all turning fifty in 2008. Peggy was first, in January, followed by Terry B., me, Debbie, Helen, Mary C., Terry S., and, finally, Mary A. (a.k.a. "Madam"). I have known Mary A. and Terry B. since I was seven years old. I met Helen in high school at age fourteen, and the others I met when I was eighteen and we had a summerhouse together in Margate, New Jersey.

Our group is affectionately known as the "Hens." (There are actually two more hens—Mary Kay and Pam—but they had already turned the magic number of fifty and were not up for re-celebrating.) There's another very close friend I must mention, even though she was not part of the "Hen" group—my friend Mary Liz, who I've known since I was five years old. She also turned fifty that year, but she had her hands full with her family and siblings' families. (She is one of ten children!) Finally, my friend Maureen, who is a few years younger than all of us, but recently joined the fifties club. (She's still a kid!)

The reason I mention the "Hens" and "almost Hens" is that these wonderful women have been part of my life for over forty years—some even longer. No matter what changes our bodies have gone through over the years, it never matters to the "Hens." We are who we are, and everyone has always been loving and accepting of each other. We are not the type of women who have ever cared about the latest fashion trends, how much money someone makes, or where they live. You'll never meet a more down-to-earth, fun group of women, and that's what makes them so special.

So we decided to go to Las Vegas to celebrate our fiftieth birthdays. I had planned to get in shape months beforehand, but, as usual, it didn't happen quite the way I envisioned. I went to the gym and tried to make healthy eating choices, but let's just say my goal of dropping thirty pounds was way off—by about twenty-five pounds. Still, I thought I looked at least halfway decent—I had shaped up the jiggly arms somewhat and shaved some tonnage off my midsection. I poured myself into my stretchy one-piece bathing suit, donned an attractive beach cover-up, and headed to the pool.

There I was poolside at Caesar's Palace, sipping a fifteen-dollar piña colada and basking my bodice in the sun. I was feeling pretty damn good at that point—even smug—until I realized I was sitting right next to Debbie in her size two bikini.

At fifty, Debbie had—and still has to this day—the stomach of a nineteen-year-old. The last time I saw clothes that small they were on my Barbie doll. I tried to shoo her away, but it wasn't working. I briefly considered jamming her into a duffle bag and heaving it onto Las Vegas Boulevard, but that wouldn't have been nice. She's still my friend, so instead I turned to her as she lounged in her teeny green bikini and gave her a big smile.

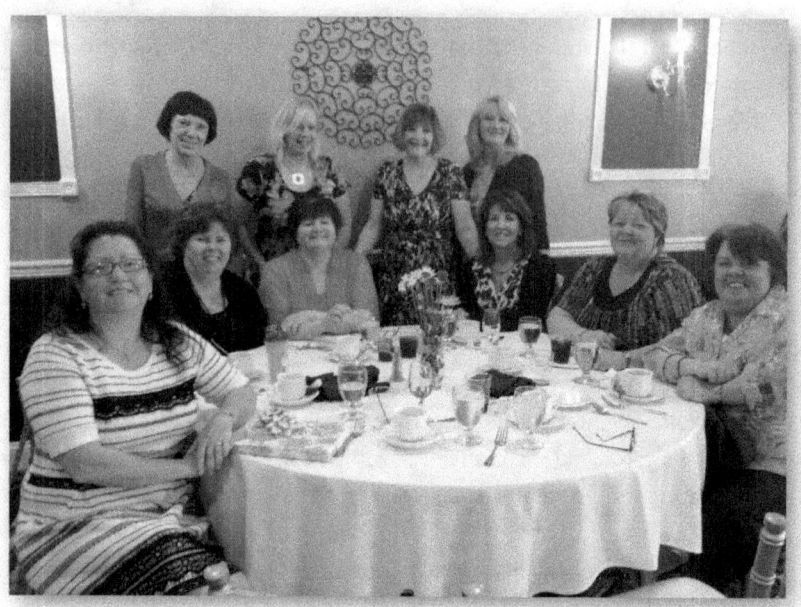

The "Hens" at Maureen's bridal shower in Drexel Hill, PA, 2014
Standing, from left: Terri B., Me, Helen, and Mary Kay
Sitting, from left: Maureen, Terry S, Mary C., Debbie, Peggy, and Madam

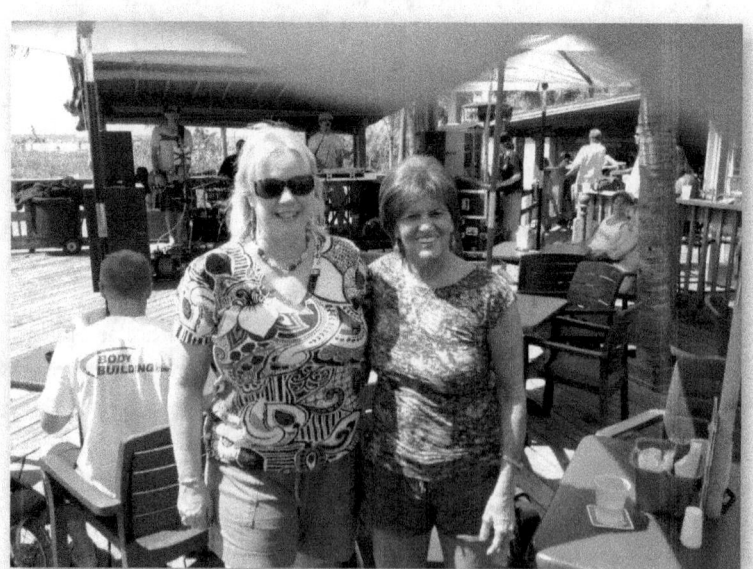

From left, Me and Pam in Tampa, FL, 2012

The rest of our vacation was an eating fest and an amazing discovery of a new elixir called the Italian margarita. It was also a grim reality check that I was, in fact, fifty years old, and there was not a damn thing I could do about it. It was a setback of sorts, but we were so happy and having so much fun, it didn't matter.

One night, after attending a Barry Manilow concert (a dead giveaway that we weren't twenty anymore), we decided to go to one of those fancy Las Vegas dance clubs. A taxi driver had given us free passes for the club, and we figured, what the hell? (He probably thought the joke would be on the club owners, as we were definitely the oldest ones there. Those club owners had probably done something to piss off that cabbie, and this was his way of getting back at them.)

We lined up out outside the club with the "kids"—the girls in thigh-high skirts and sky-high heels, and the guys in silk shirts unbuttoned to the navel. When the time came for our grand entry, a kid at the door asked me for ID. (Was he blind?) I politely told the kid I was fifty, that he had to be joking, and that I didn't have any ID with me. In a flash, a large bouncer headed toward us, flashlight in hand. (The club was dark.) He took one look at us and showed us right in. There was absolutely no question that we were old enough.

Once inside, we made a beeline for the back of the club and stood there laughing. Debbie claimed she had heard someone call her "grandma," and then she started kvetching that the place was too cold. (That's one good thing about having extra weight—the fat keeps you warm.) We refused to allow her to put on her sweater, fearing it would call even more attention to the "old broads in the back."

After about a half hour, we bailed. We were glad to get out of there, and I'm sure the rest of the pubescent population was as well. If there was any question as to whether we looked our age, it was answered that night.

The next night, however, we were vindicated. At a concert featuring The Coasters, The Platters, and The Temptations, we were among the youngest in the audience. We loved it! Not only was the music fantastic, but we were once again the "kids." (Of course, being the "kids" at our sixtieth and seventieth birthday celebrations might prove difficult if we can't find enough people in their eighties and nineties. Well, we'll just worry about that later.)

The next few years were hit or miss—mostly miss—until I discovered that setbacks are a part of life and I was going to have to deal with them. Life is a series of ups and downs—joy and sadness. I learned that when bad or unexpected things happen, it's OK to let myself screw up and get off track for a while.

My cat Muffin died of cancer at the age of fourteen and, again, it was another loss in my life. Some months later, I adopted Oliver, a tiny ten-week-old kitten. He and Melody, my "baby girl" adopted in 2007, were like typical brothers and sisters—fighting one minute and playing the next.

Perhaps one of the greatest losses in my life came in December of 2015 when I lost my best friend, Mary A. (aka "Madam"). We had known each other since we were seven years old. Losing your parents is devastating enough, but having a friend you have known for fifty-one years pass away is just beyond comprehension. Because her death was so sudden—a tragic car accident—dealing with it has been very difficult, even now.

I dedicated this book to Madam, as we spent years lamenting about weight gain, flabby guts, wiggly arms, thunderous thighs, and rotund rear ends. I miss our crazy conversations that often began with things like, "I'm so fat that I'm being featured at the whaling museum," or, "I'm so fat that I'm being hired as the next Goodyear blimp."

We met in elementary school and had been best friends ever since. We went through everything together—her first boyfriend, my first boyfriend, her first marriage, and my first (and only) marriage. I was her maid of honor and she was mine. We helped each other through our divorces. Later, when she married Joe, I was her matron of honor. Neither of us had children, and we were both fine with that.

We both had unrealistic fears of the dentist and often shared horror stories of being drilled. The only thing we feared worse than the dentist was the gynecologist. We would try to outdo each other with frightening tales of being spread-eagle on the table with our feet in the stirrups, and the finale of the exam with the gruesome anal cavity check. There are not many people with whom you can share your most disgusting memories, and I was lucky to have Madam as my confidant. Perhaps most bizarre, we'd often talk about death and what would happen if we were pushing one hundred and lost control of our bowels. We both agreed that, at this point, we would shoot each other. Now, I suppose, I'll have to find someone else to pull the trigger.

When we were in high school, we spent hours on the phone, and often my mom would pick up the receiver downstairs at my house and say, "She's *still* on!" Once we took her brother's car for a wild ride and got it stuck in the mud. We had to call a tow truck to get it out.

Madam, Helen, and I were in the high school orchestra together—we all played the violin. One day the three of us were in the music room trying out other instruments, and Madam got stuck in a tuba. We managed to get her out with no injuries.

Madam and I took our first trip out of the country—to Bermuda—when we were eighteen. We met a cast of characters, rode mopeds wearing Batgirl helmets, and ended up at some British woman's party with a live band and really crappy food.

In our early twenties, we shared a room in our Margate summerhouse with the rest of the "Hens." Mom and Aunt Tiny called our rental home "The Flophouse"; it really was a dump, but we loved it. We drank beer and ate pizza, but Madam would eat only the pizza crusts. She didn't like the rest of it. Sometimes early in the morning, after the bars had closed, we'd have pizza then throw pizza crusts into our room for her after Madam had gone to bed. Bizarre, I know.

After I moved to New York in my late twenties, we didn't see each other as much, but talked constantly on the phone. Sometimes, we'd spend hours talking about nonsense, which was perfectly normal for us. When we did see each other, it was a laugh-fest no matter what we talked about. We both loved disco dancing and would call each other without fail when "Heaven Must Be Missing An Angel" came on the radio.

We spent many summers at the New Jersey shore and, more recently, at Cape Cod where Madam literally split her pants laughing. I can't remember what we were laughing at, though. It was probably something childish or ridiculous, but it didn't matter. We thought it was funny.

On our birthdays, she would always serenade each of the "Hens" with her own special rendition of "Happy Birthday," and if we were really lucky, we'd also get an encore performance of "On the Way to Cape May." During those times when she'd had a bit too much to drink, we would be treated to songs like "High Hopes" and her Frank Sinatra favorite, "Summer Wind."

The last time I saw her was August 2015 at my friend Terry S.'s summerhouse in Sea Isle City, New Jersey. We did the beach, shopping, and then headed out to an early afternoon oldies show with Jerry Blavat, the famous Philadelphia DJ and TV personality. Anyone from Philly also knows him as "The Geator with the Heater" and the "Boss with the Hot Sauce." (I think Helen still has a crush on him.)

When Madam and I were Girl Scouts, we got the chance to be in the studio audience of "The Jerry Blavat Show" in Philadelphia. We were starstruck, and his special musical guest, Billy Harner, sang his hit "Sally Saying Something." (Yeah, we're old!) Fast-forward to our last summer together in 2015—we had a grand old time eating, dancing, and laughing, and it was the first time in a long while that many of the "Hens" had been together. I'm so glad the last time I saw her was such a memorable experience.

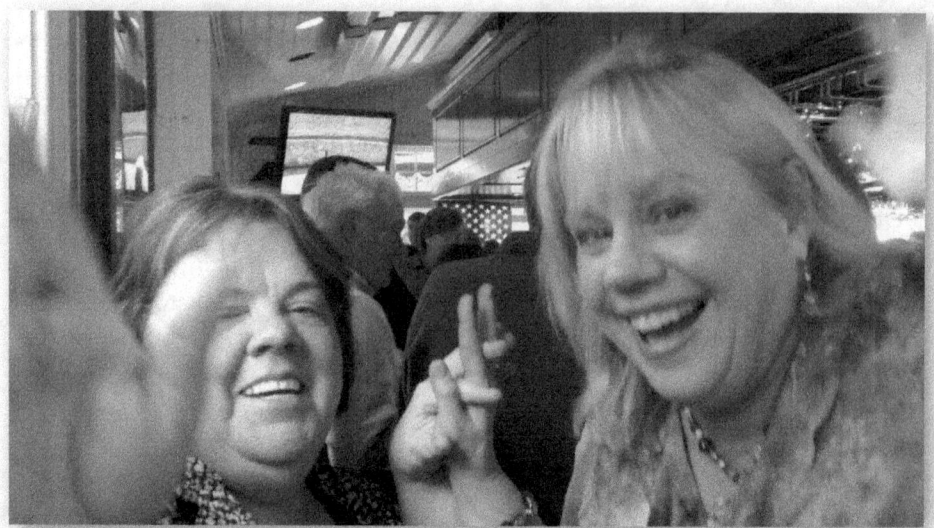

From left, Madam and Me dancing in Cape Cod, MA, 2013

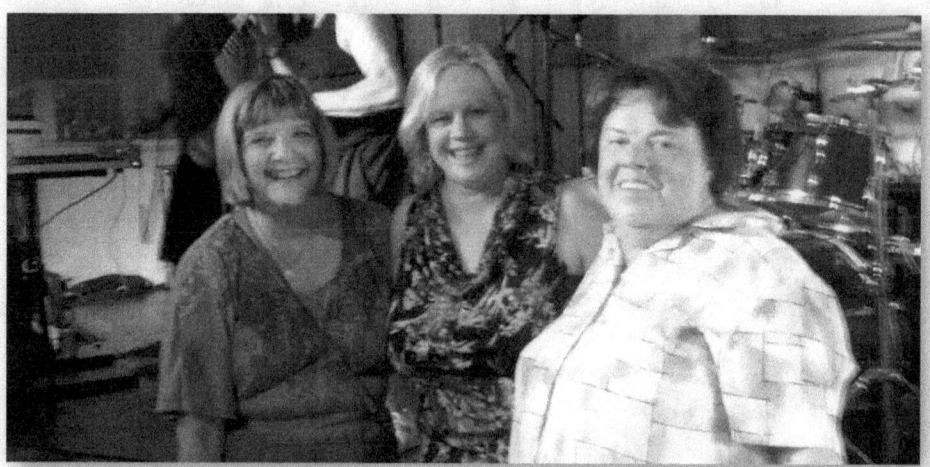

From left, Helen, Me and Madam in Sea Isle City, NJ, 2015 This was the last time I saw Madam.

What's very strange is that the year before Madam's death, we both were making progress in dropping the pounds. I had joined the new Wellness Club at the hospital that was my saving grace, and she had started walking and eating healthier.

After she passed, for the very first time I didn't go into "setback mode." When I returned home after the funeral in Pennsylvania, I didn't take any time off from the gym and continued to eat healthy. At that point, I was down to 179 pounds—a number I hadn't seen in years. The fact that I had made it past 190, and even 180, encouraged me to stay focused. I also think Madam would have been angry with me if I had let my sadness act as a setback. In the back of my mind, I could hear her saying, "OK, so just because I died, you're going to slack off? Well, you're not blaming me if you get fat!"

I've talked about a lot of setbacks that I experienced over the years and about how I failed to deal with them. I've had nineteen years to think about this and have come to the simple conclusion that life is always going to have some bad times, sadness, and disappointments. Dealing with them isn't easy, and I'm not going to pretend that it is.

My most recent setback was the passing of yet another one of my fur babies. Melody was just about ten years old and suffered for about a year with a liver disease. She survived surgery and seemed to be heading toward recovery, but then took a turn for the worse. Her death made me think once more about everyone I've lost—my parents, Aunt Tiny and Madam.

I will leave you with one really funny, memorable setback which happened just prior to publishing this book – in December 2017. I had to add this because I wanted to end this chapter on a happy note.

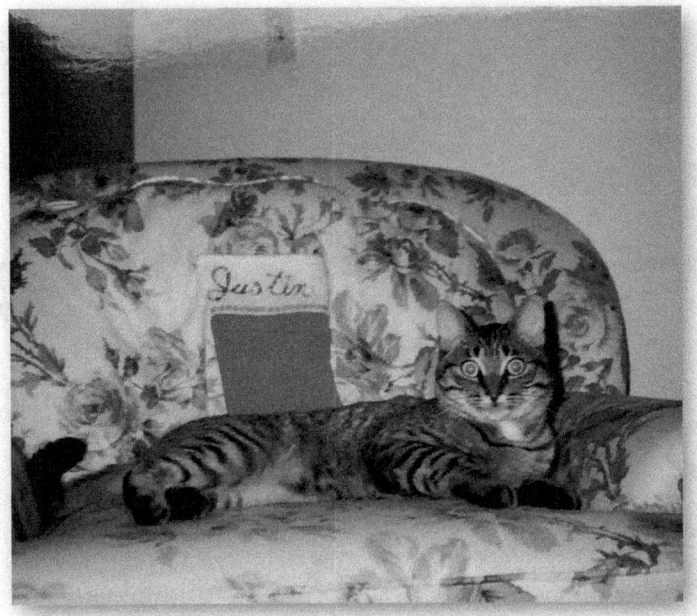

Justin Prenon, 1999 – 2007

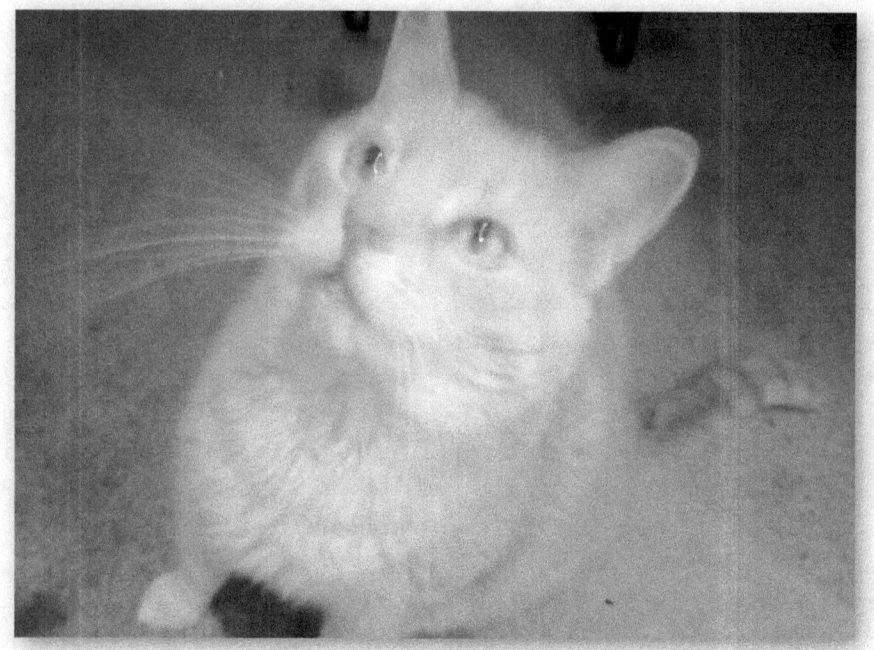

Muffin Prenon, 2001 - 2013

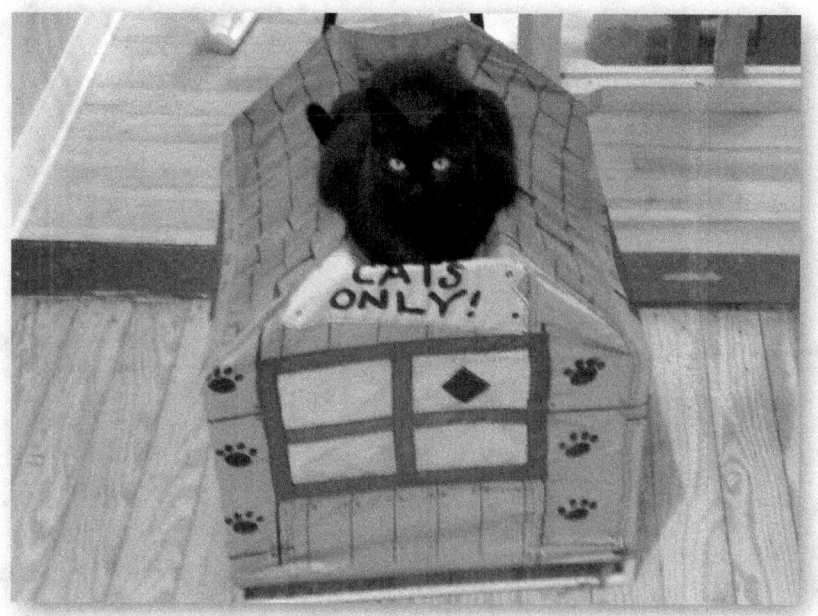

Melody Prenon, 2007- 2017

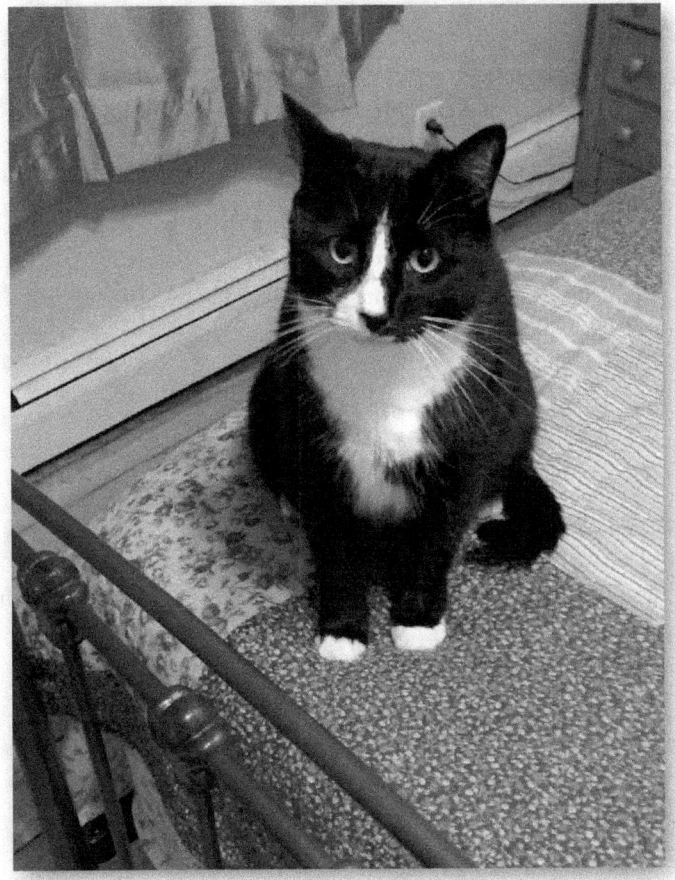

Oliver Prenon, 2013 - present

I'm calling it the "Prenon Christmas Catastrophe." As I've stated many times, a gourmet cook I am not. If it wasn't for the outdoor grill, my George Foreman griller and my microwave, I'd probably starve to death. Anyhow, in a moment of sheer madness, I agreed to host Christmas dinner at my house, where I would be cooking the turkey (actually a turkey breast, but still a damn big meal).

I awoke early Christmas morning, gave Oliver his presents – a myriad of toy mice – and began to prepare the grub. I made a lovely vegetarian dish for my friend JoEllen's daughter Christina (very easy – quinoa, beans and tomatoes in one pan), salad (you can't mess that up – just toss in a few bags of veggies), and vegetarian "meat" balls (thrown in the microwave with tomato sauce from a jar.) The rest of the "trimmings" would be microwaveable frozen veggies and some Pepperidge Farm stuffing from JoEllen.

Just as I was preparing to place the bird in the oven, I noticed a weird code on the oven keypad. I started pre-heating it at 325, but now there was just a strange "7" appearing. When I pushed the "off" button, there was no response. After several more pushes and a few choice words, I scrambled to find the oven manual and see just what the hell was going on. I looked through the troubleshooting section and nada.

The hilarity continued as I frantically flew to the basement, switching circuit breaker after circuit breaker, trying to shut down the damn oven. (Of course, the rooms and appliances were not accurately marked on the inside of the breaker box!) When I finally found the correct one, the stove quietly died. And it remained dead after flipping the breaker back on.

Next came the near hysterical call to JoEllen, seeking a place to cook the bird. Alas, her oven had been broken for years -- she relies on her stovetop and griller for meal preparation. Another frenzied call was placed to my neighbor, Sharon, who was outside shoveling snow and didn't get the call.

So, there I sat, screaming, crying, and then laughing about the fact that my oven chose Christmas Day to go on strike. I concluded that this was my payback for not using it enough over the years. The vile appliance had probably been plotting this for weeks!

Fortunately, I ran into Sharon outside and she gladly offered not only her oven, but her home for hosting Christmas dinner. (Ironically, we had all been at her home for dessert on Christmas Eve, after having dinner together at a local restaurant.)

While I was disappointed that I would no longer be hosting the soiree (I had even set the table with china and a tablecloth), I was elated that we would not be forced to chomp into a raw turkey for dinner.

That "Kodak moment" came as I whisked the turkey across our rather lengthy snow-covered lawns to Sharon's house! Equally as "picture-perfect" a scene was me schlepping a five-pound bag of potatoes and a bottle of wine across the lawn.

My whole point in recounting this story is to let you know that after settling into Sharon's home on "turkey watch," I proceeded to make a beeline for the chocolate cookies and brownies on her kitchen counter. After the ordeal I had been through, all of my healthy eating habits flew out the window.

The dinner turned out great, the bird was fabulous and a good time was had by all. Of course, dessert followed and I helped myself to apple pie, cheesecake and some more cookies.

While I had planned to "cheat" just a bit on Christmas on the whole healthy thing, I had gone completely overboard. The important thing is that I didn't let my one day of "setback eating" dictate my dietary behavior for the rest of the week. The next day, I was back munching salads again and going to the gym that night after work. (Incidentally, I was the ONLY one at the Wellness Club that night! Just saying!)

So, the big question is -- Will all of the stressful times we experience always result in setbacks in healthy eating and exercising? No, but they will happen. Here's the thing—if you go into this knowing you will probably screw up sometimes, that's half the battle. Forgive yourself for screwing up, and then get back on track as soon as possible.

My problem had always been that I didn't forgive myself. I continued to get angry with myself, which led to being depressed about my weight, which led to overeating and under-exercising. I finally learned to stop and say, "OK, so what? So I made a pig of myself, gained a few extra pounds, feel like crap, and look even worse. So what?!" Then, without thinking about it anymore, I moved on.

What Works for Me in Dealing with Setbacks

1. Stop thinking about it! You messed up—big deal. Don't give it one more thought. Start the next day fresh and to hell with your screwup.
2. Take a walk. (Now, this may not be possible if it's midnight and you're in a crying fit. However, you can plan a walk for the following day.)
3. Call a friend and lament. Believe me, this always helps.
4. Listen to some soft music and clear your mind.
5. Eat something healthy like a piece of fruit or a vegetable. This will help to get you in the right frame of mind.
6. Do a plank position. It will help tighten your core and get your mind and body ready for the next day.
7. Do some arm or leg exercises while watching TV.
8. Try some deep breathing. This will relax you and get you out of your funk.
9. Go for a manicure or pedicure. (Again, this may not be possible if it's the middle of the night. Unless, of course, you know someone offering "emergency" manicures!)
10. This one is reserved for those really bad moments, and I guarantee you will feel absolutely wonderful afterward. Take one of those skinny model catalogs, throw it in the trash, and then toss cat poop on top of it. I've actually

done this after cleaning out the cats' litter boxes. Pitch the poop right on top of that size four. (If you don't have a cat, you can use garbage like banana peels, egg shells, etc. It may not have the same impact as the cat crap, but it will still make you feel better.)

CHAPTER 7

Maintaining it All

Well, now that you're motivated, exercising, eating healthy, and dealing with setbacks, how do you maintain it all? Beats the hell out of me! I have to be honest—I can't tell you exactly how to maintain your healthy weight, because I don't have a very good track record for that.

As I've stated many times throughout this book, I have struggled with my weight my entire adult life and will have to constantly be mindful of how much I'm exercising and eating every day for the rest of my life.

What seems to be working for me is making exercise a priority in my life. I head to the Wellness Club every day after work. (I don't go home first, because once I'm home, I know I'm not going back out again.) Sometimes, when the weather is really nice, I'll walk outside at a local park for up to an hour. My Fitbit keeps track of my steps, and I strive to reach my ten thousand-step goal every day. On Saturdays and Sundays, I'll walk outside. Almost every day I log my food choices into My Fitness Pal. Sometimes it's a pain in the butt; however, at this point, I'm so used to doing it that it's almost second nature. In fact, the few times that I don't log in my food, it feels weird, like I'm missing out on something.

After breaking through each weight milestone, I promised myself I would do whatever it takes (with the exception of diet pills, powders, and any other unnatural crap) to prevent the scale from going up again.

What's very strange for me right now is that my body is finally in a healthy weight zone and most of my clothes are too big. Of course, I can't afford to buy a whole new wardrobe, so I'm wearing those formerly too-fat-to-fit-into clothes that somehow miraculously fit. I have started shopping a bit, and for the first time in about twenty years, I'm trying on sizes ten and twelve. (Note: some of those "oh-so-skinny" clothing stores will have you believe that a size twelve, fourteen, and even sixteen are plus sizes. Just for the record, that is total bullshit!)

So, what exactly is a "healthy weight"? Well, it depends on your sex, height, age, and body type. Men typically weigh more than women, so if you're a guy, you're in luck. There are many different weight charts out there—some are accurate, and some are completely ridiculous. (Remember the idiots at that now-defunct weight loss center who told me my ideal weight was 135?!)

I've looked at many weight range charts, and one of the most accurate is the Weight Watchers chart. I have a medium to large frame and am fairly muscular and now sixty years old. The top of the weight range for me is 160, which is also the number my cardiologist recommended.

I don't know what my all-time-high weight was because, for the longest time, I refused to step on a scale. The highest number I ever saw was 198, but I know I exceeded that when I could barely squeeze into my size sixteen clothes. If I had to guess, I'd say I hit the top probably around 210.

It took me a total of nineteen years to drop those fifty pounds because I kept losing and gaining back the same 20 pounds all the time. (Just call me "Miss Yoyo"). I should have been able to do it much quicker but again, I'm lazy, and I love to eat!

When I first broke 190 pounds, it was a joy and a curse at the same time. I'd been able to accomplish this several times over the years, but never managed to get below 183. Then a setback would happen. I'd get lazy, and, sooner or later, I'd be back at 190 or more. I can't tell you how many times I repeated that scenario over the years.

When I joined the Wellness Club in January 2015, I was hovering at about 195 pounds. The thing that kept me going all this time was not giving up. I didn't care if it took me until I was ninety-five years old—I was going to get healthy again. I set out to do this, and I was going to do it no matter how difficult it was or how long it took.

The Wellness Club was the right fit for me. This small, friendly place was so welcoming that I began to look forward to going there instead of dreading it. As I started to see small results—a bit less muffin top and jiggling of my thighs—I started to make healthier eating choices. I didn't want to destroy all the hard work I had done.

Within several months, I was elated to see the scale reporting 182 pounds—a number I hadn't seen in twelve years. Then the summer came, and while I wasn't as active as I should have been, I did maintain the weight. By November, I had accomplished the impossible—I broke 180. It took a hell of a long time, but by the end of 2015, the scale had stopped at 175.

For the first time in my adult life, I was starting a new year at a half-decent weight. I made a new commitment to myself, worked out longer and harder, and made a conscious effort to watch my sodium intake after those nasty AFib incidents. In only five months I had done the unthinkable—broken 170. My weight in April 2016 was 167.

While I was determined to reach my goal weight by the beginning of the summer, it just didn't' happen. In fact, I was stuck at 167 for almost another year. No matter what I did, the scale would not move. I tried walking more and eating less, but nothing worked. I was stuck. Maybe this is as far as I'm supposed to get, I thought.

However, I was hell bent on dropping the final seven pounds, so I did the unthinkable—I went back to Zumba class! Now, I must mention again how physically uncoordinated I am, so this was an extreme challenge. I had been to Zumba off and on over the past couple of years—more off than on. The good thing was that most of the people in the class were over fifty—the bad thing was that I still couldn't keep up with them! The first few times were truly exhausting and embarrassing. My feet were going in all different directions, and when the class moved one way across the floor, I was moving the other way. Sure, I love to dance—but at my own pace and using my own simple choreography.

Never one to quit, I stuck with it, and while there are a few Zumba dances that my feet will never quite understand, I'm in it for the long haul. It's also a great way to get your steps in. One class usually clocks over five thousand steps!

Finally, by the summer of 2017, I had painstakingly lost the final seven pounds and reached my goal of 160 by my 60th birthday. Those last few pounds were a nightmare to lose—getting in my ten thousand steps almost every day and being very conscious of eating only healthy food. After a while though, I got careless and of course, the pounds starting to grow back. I found myself back in the same situation again, watching the scale sway from 166 to 167.

So in addition to the eating healthy, exercising and Zumba, I decided I had to add some interval training. I'm not a runner, but I started running for about five minutes at a time on the treadmill, then resumed walking for another five to ten minutes, then running again for a few minutes and so on. (I'm not talking marathon running here -- I'm talking a light jog, but it still does the trick).

By early January, I was back in the 160 zone, and determined more than ever to stop that damn scale from taunting me again with its hideous 160-plus numbers. From now on, the numbers can go only south!

The bottom line is that for the rest of my life, I'll have to continuously watch my food intake and get in enough exercise to maintain a healhty weight. (I've found that the elliptical machine is a great calorie killer, and twenty to thirty minutes works wonders). Despite the fact that this whole healthy living thing can still totally suck, for the first time in my life, I'm really happy with my weight!

Perhaps the biggest positive change I've experienced is the ability to say "no" to the free junk food that confronts me at just about every networking event I attend—and there are tons and tons of events. It's always the same thing—fried chicken wings, fried mozzarella sticks, fried tater tots or facsimile, and nasty pasta. Would it kill them to put out some fresh vegetables?

Years ago I would have dived headfirst into the appetizers and come up for air only to have a swig of beer. Now the thought of eating that type of food completely freaks me out for two reasons—one is my fear of hidden "sodium bombs" triggering an "AFib" episode, and the other is the fear of Dr. K. beating the crap out of me for gaining the weight back! No seriously, I have just lost interest in unhealthy eating. I've worked so hard for so many years to get where I am, and I'll do anything in my power to keep from reverting back to a grossly overweight, high-blood-pressure, high-cholesterol being.

I recently saw Dr. K.—the same man who seven years ago told me I was "heavy." The first words out of his mouth this time were, "You look great." (Just a minute, Doc. Can I get a video of that, please?) I think he was even happier than I was with my new weight of 160. The other good news is that my cholesterol numbers are the best they have been in years, and Dr. K. has given the OK for me to come off the medication! As for the blood pressure meds, no such luck. That's OK, because I'm on a low dose beta blocker that also helps with the Afib. No biggie!

So what does the future hold? Hell if I know. Could I end up gaining the weight back? Yes, I could, if I'm not careful. Could I lose more? Maybe, but I'm going to take what life gives me. If I maintain, great, and if I can drop to 155, I'll definitely alert the media. My approach is to take it just one day at a time.

Every day will continue to be a challenge for me. I've never been a naturally thin person (except for infancy), so I constantly have to think about what I'm eating, record what I'm eating, and, most importantly, exercise.

Sometimes that sucks, but I have to be realistic and look at this whole thing as a positive, not a negative. I'm healthier than I've been in many years, and I finally feel good about the way I look. You can't ask for more than that. So, if I have to "suck it up" by eating healthy and exercising, then that's what I'll continue to do.

Sure, we're all going to croak someday, but let's keep the Grim Reaper at bay for as long as we can! Making healthy food choices and exercise a part of your life can actually be pretty cool because it makes you stronger both physically and mentally. (And it will keep you dancing well into your 90's and beyond!) After nineteen years, I finally get it!

What Works for Me in Maintaining a Healthy Weight

1. Record what you eat. It sucks in the beginning, but believe me it's worth it. Use one of the many free smartphone apps like My Fitness Pal.
2. Do some type of exercise at least five days a week. If you're really busy, it can just be a short walk. Keeping active is the key.
3. Don't drive yourself crazy with the scale. Weigh yourself once a week. I usually like to do it on Friday mornings. It's before the weekend, when many people tend to stray from their healthy program a bit. Also, weigh yourself naked. You don't want to add any extra pounds. (Make sure the window shades are down when you're doing this!)
4. If you find that you have gained back a pound or two, don't freak out. Commit to stepping up the workouts the following week, and keep your hands out of the cookie jar!
5. Read health-related articles. Google anything to do with healthy weight, and you'll find lots of great information to help you maintain.

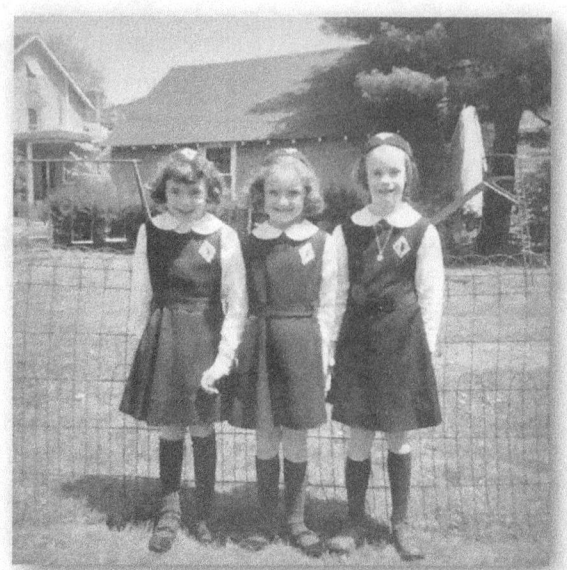

From left, Terry B, Mary Liz and Me in my yard in Drexel Hill, PA at 6 years old, 1963

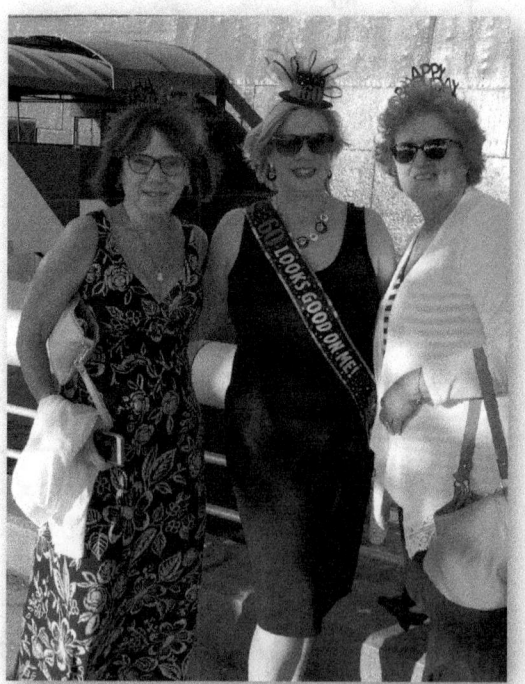

From left, Terry B, Me and Mary Liz at 60 years old at my 60th Birthday
Celebration in downtown Philadelphia, PA, 2017

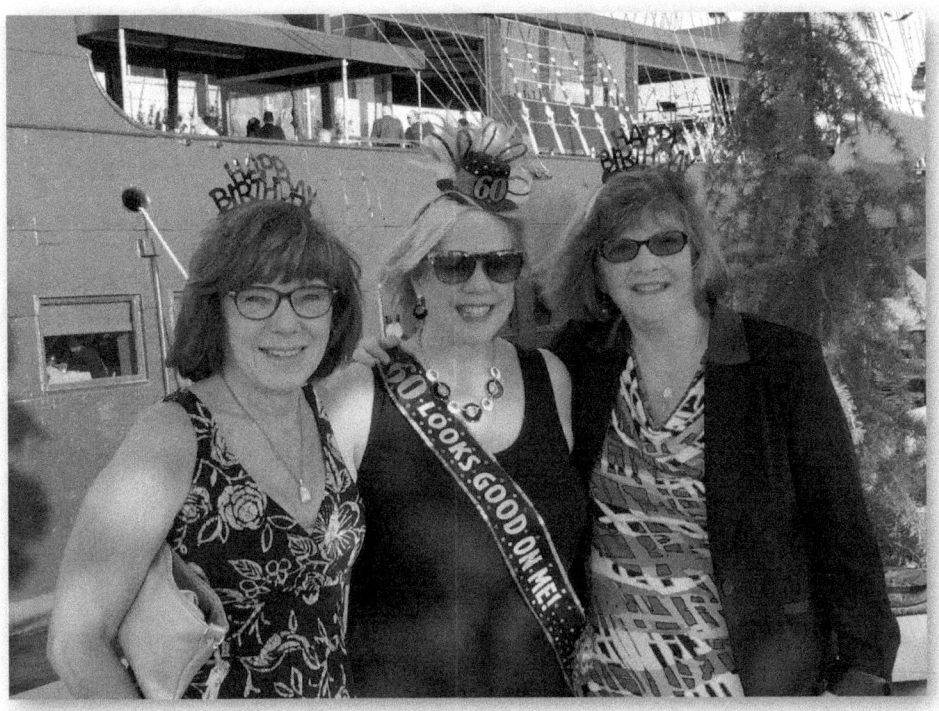

From left, Terry B, Me, and Helen at my 60th Birthday Celebration in downtown Philadelphia, PA, 2017

CHAPTER 8

Mary's Daily Menu Suggestions (and Idiot-Proof Healthy Recipes)

The last thing I want to do is make this so difficult and time consuming that you give up before you start. Many "diet" books have long, complicated recipes, and when you work all day then get home from the gym at seven-thirty at night, who the hell has time to prepare elaborate meals?

Also, please keep in mind that these are only my suggestions. Dr. K and some dietitians may disagree with some of my choices, but these are ones that have worked for me. I'll keep this as simple as possible because, truthfully, I'm still kind of lazy!

At the end of these suggestions, you'll find a brief list of basic kitchen equipment and groceries.

Breakfast Suggestions

Greek Yogurt Smoothie

1. Throw 0 percent plain Greek yogurt (I like Fage—low sugar, low sodium and high protein) and fruit into a blender with water and some ice.
2. Blend and drink.

Eggs and Omelets

1. Crack open two eggs, and throw them into frying pan. (Use Pam spray instead of butter.)

2. Eat. (If you have high cholesterol, eat eggs only a couple times a week.)

Fruit

1. Choose low-sugar fruits like berries, melons, apples, or kiwi. Bananas are higher in sugar but are a good source of potassium.
2. Eat.

Oatmeal

1. Look for low-carb and low-sugar varieties.
2. Add boiling water, sir and eat.

English Muffins, Waffles, or Pancakes

1. Eat only low-carb varieties, maybe one or two days a week. Throw on some peanut butter for protein. Don't combine with bagels!

Bagels

1. Don't eat unless you're suffering horribly from a bagel craving. Then eat a maximum of one per week when you get to your goal weight.

Pastries, Croissants, and Sticky Buns

1. Run from!

Lunch Suggestions
Salads with Protein

1. Buy a bag of salad, and throw some grilled chicken, turkey, or shrimp on it. (Grill several chicken breasts on Sundays so you can "grab and go" for the week.)
2. Go to a salad bar, but lay off the cheese, cranberries, eggs, and bacon bits.
3. Eat.

Lettuce Wraps

1. Use iceberg, romaine, or Bibb lettuce as the "bread" and stuff with chicken, turkey, or another choice of protein. Throw in some tomatoes, sprouts, cucumbers, peppers, etc.
2. Eat.

Fresh Veggies and Hummus

1. Buy sliced peppers, carrots, broccoli, snap peas, cauliflower, celery, tomatoes, or other fresh veggies.
2. Dip in low-sodium, low-fat hummus.
3. Eat.

Tomato and Tuna or Chicken Salad

1. Slice a large tomato, leaving it intact at the bottom, and then throw either chicken or tuna salad in the middle. (Better to make the chicken or tuna salad yourself using low-fat mayo.)
2. Eat.

Soup

1. Buy low-sodium soup (I like Health Valley) in the organic section of the grocery store.
2. Microwave and eat.

Veggie Burgers

1. Microwave and eat.

Dinner Leftovers

2. Microwave and eat.

Sandwiches

1. Buy or make a chicken, turkey, roast beef, or veggie sandwich at least once a week so you won't get sick of salads. Go for multigrain bread.
2. Eat.

Sushi

1. Buy and eat. (I like only the vegetable sushi. Choose the brown rice ones over the white rice.)

If you want something else to go with your lunch, like chips, there are healthy selections out there. Again, I'm spoiled because Whole Foods is located downstairs in our office building, and there are tons of different choices for chips. I like the purple chips or rice chips. I always look for sodium levels no greater than 150. Look for brands that offer you the most amount of chips for the least amount of calories or sodium. Some types let you have up to fifteen chips. Yes, I do count them out. I know—it's kind of depressing, but it will keep you from consuming the entire bag!

Dinner Suggestions

Roasted Chicken Dinner

1. Buy a precooked chicken at the grocery store, a sweet potato or boil-in-bag brown rice, and either fresh or frozen veggies (no sauce).
2. Microwave or boil the frozen veggies, and throw your boil-in-bag brown rice in boiling water.
3. Eat.

Grilled Chicken Dinner

1. Throw chicken on a George Foreman griller or on an outdoor grill. Garnish with any type of low-sugar, low-sodium sauce.
2. Microwave or boil the veggies.
3. Eat.

Chicken or Fish in a Wok Dinner

1. Cut up chicken, and throw in wok with olive oil and cook. (Or you can use shrimp or scallops.)
2. Throw in a bag of fresh veggies, and garnish with any type of low-sugar, low-sodium sauce.
3. Throw a boil-in-bag of brown rice in boiling water.
4. Eat.

Baked Chicken Dinner

1. Throw chicken in a pan with any type of low-sugar, low-sodium sauce, and bake.
2. Microwave or boil some veggies.
3. Eat.

Baked or Grilled Fish Dinner

1. Throw fish on the grill or in the oven with any type of low-sugar, low-sodium sauce.
2. Microwave or boil some veggies.
3. Eat.

Stuffed Peppers

1. Cook ground turkey or beef with some low-sodium tomato sauce.
2. Slice the top off a bell pepper and fill with the meat sauce.
3. Eat.

Veggie Pasta

1. Buy premade zucchini or butternut squash "pasta," and boil.
2. Throw on some protein of your choice with low-sodium sauce.
3. Eat.

Veggie Burgers

1. Buy frozen veggie burgers and microwave.
2. Eat.

I'm a chicken, turkey, and fish kind of person, but you can also throw some burgers on the grill as well. I don't like steak, duck, lamb, veal, or pork, so I can't give you any suggestions there. I eat roast beef occasionally, but haven't the slightest idea how to roast a beef. (Mom would not be happy. She spent hours trying to show me how to cook a roast beef.)

If you're a vegetarian, you can always Google "easy vegetarian recipes." I've found several really easy ones.

Snack Suggestions

Apples and Peanut Butter

1. Cut up an apple and slather with peanut butter.
2. Eat.

Zucchini Nachos

1. Arrange sliced zucchini rounds on a plate, and cover with low-sodium salsa and low-sodium Mexican cheese.
2. Throw in microwave for about two minutes.
3. Eat.

Veggies

1. Buy sliced peppers, carrots, broccoli, snap peas, cauliflower, celery, tomatoes, or other fresh veggies.
2. Dip in low-sodium, low-fat hummus.
3. Eat.

Popcorn

1. Look for low-sodium "ready to eat" varieties in individual packs. (I like Skinny Pop.)
2. Tear open one pack.
3. Eat.

Nuts

1. Buy the unsalted kind—almonds, mixed nuts, walnuts, etc.
2. Eat.

Protein Bars

1. Be very careful to buy low-sugar, low-carb bars. (I like Kind bars and Larabars).
2. Eat.

On-the-Road Food Choices

1. Salads or wraps
2. Unsalted nuts
3. Low-sugar/low-sodium protein bars
4. Fruit
5. Yogurt (watch the sugars)
6. Peanut butter crackers (check the sodium). The peanut butter will sustain you. Crackers, not so great, but just deal with it for the day!
7. Fast food if you have to. One day is not going to kill you!

Kitchen Equipment

Here's a short list of kitchen equipment you might want to have on hand:

- BBQ grill or a George Foreman griller
- Blender
- Wok
- Veggie chopper

- Veggie pasta maker (You can find it at those As Seen on TV stores. You can turn your zucchini or other squash into "pasta" strands.)

Groceries

Here's a short list of essential grocery items:

- Greek yogurt (low sugar—I like Fage and Dannon Light & Fit)
- Fruit of any kind, but try to go for low-sugar fruits. (Enter the type of fruit into My Fitness Pal, and it will tell you the sugars.)
- Eggs
- Oatmeal (low sugar & low carb)
- English muffins (low-carb, multigrain. I like Fiber One.)
- Vegetables (any kind, fresh, frozen, and salads in a bag)
- Salad dressings and sauces (low sugar and low sodium. I like Annie's)
- Soup (low sodium—I like Healthy Valley, No Salt Added)
- Crackers (low sodium)
- Chicken breasts
- Ground turkey or ground beef
- Veggie burgers (I like Dr. Prager's)
- Fish (watch the shellfish if you're on a low-sodium diet)
- Tomato sauce and other sauces (low sodium. I like Brad's Organic)
- Brown rice (I like Success Boil-in-Bag—very quick for lazy types like me!)
- Beans (low sodium)
- Sweet potatoes
- Quinoa
- Shredded cheese (low sodium)
- Peanut butter (low sodium)
- Mayonnaise (low sodium)
- Hummus
- Unsalted nuts
- Popcorn (check the sodium—I like Skinny Pop)
- Rice crackers or any type of low-sodium crackers
- PAM spray

CHAPTER 9

Mary's Healthy Living Dos and Don'ts

First, the Don'ts

1. Don't *ever* start a healthy eating plan on a weekend.
2. Don't judge yourself against the airbrushed bodies in magazines.
3. Don't compare yourself to others. Everyone's metabolism is different.
4. Don't let other people put you down. There will always be obnoxious jerks who will try to belittle what you've accomplished. Screw them!
5. Don't get discouraged—ever! There's always tomorrow.

Now the Dos

1. Do try to be positive. I know it's damn difficult, but if you start feeling depressed, you're not going to want to do anything. Then you'll sit around and eat crap, say screw the workouts, and watch some sappy movie on Lifetime (or so I've heard).
2. Do start working out with a simple walk around the block or, when it's too cold, too hot, or raining, the mall.
3. Do at least some type of exercise every day—even if it's housework.
4. Do drink lots of water. It will fill you up and fool your stomach into thinking it's full (at least for a while).
5. Do work fruits and veggies into your everyday diet. Some days you just won't want to, but force yourself. (You'll thank yourself later.)

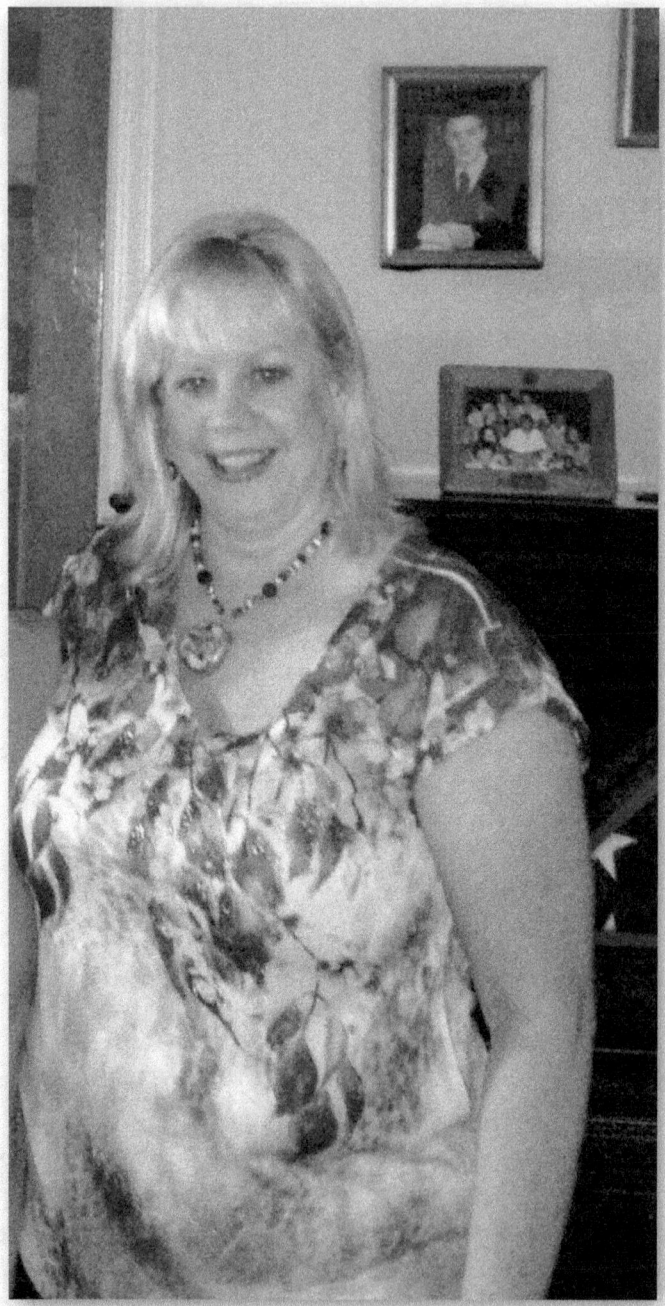

Me at 200+ Pounds at a party in Drexel Hill, PA, 2012

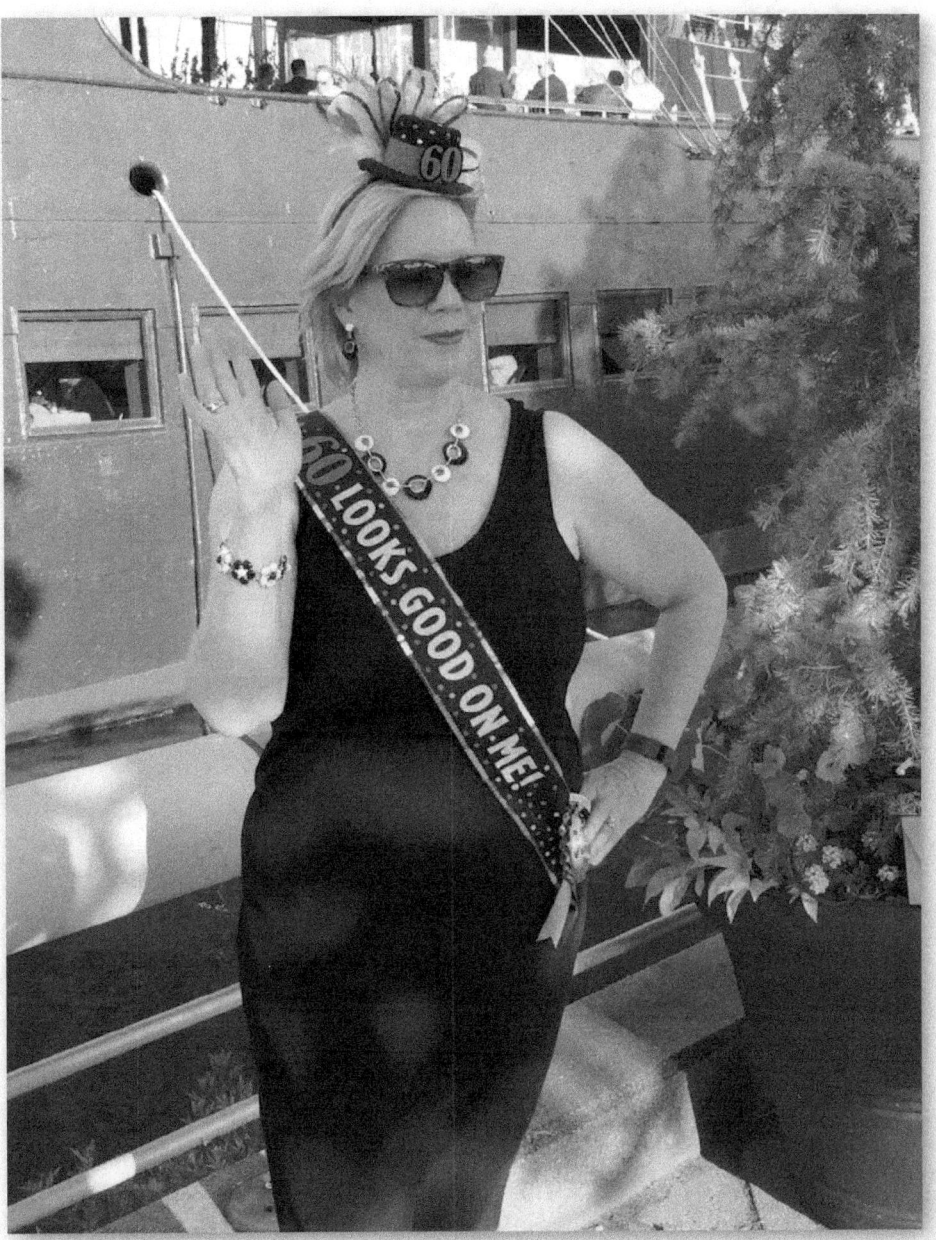

Me at 160 Pounds at my 60th Birthday Celebration in downtown Philadelphia, PA, 2017

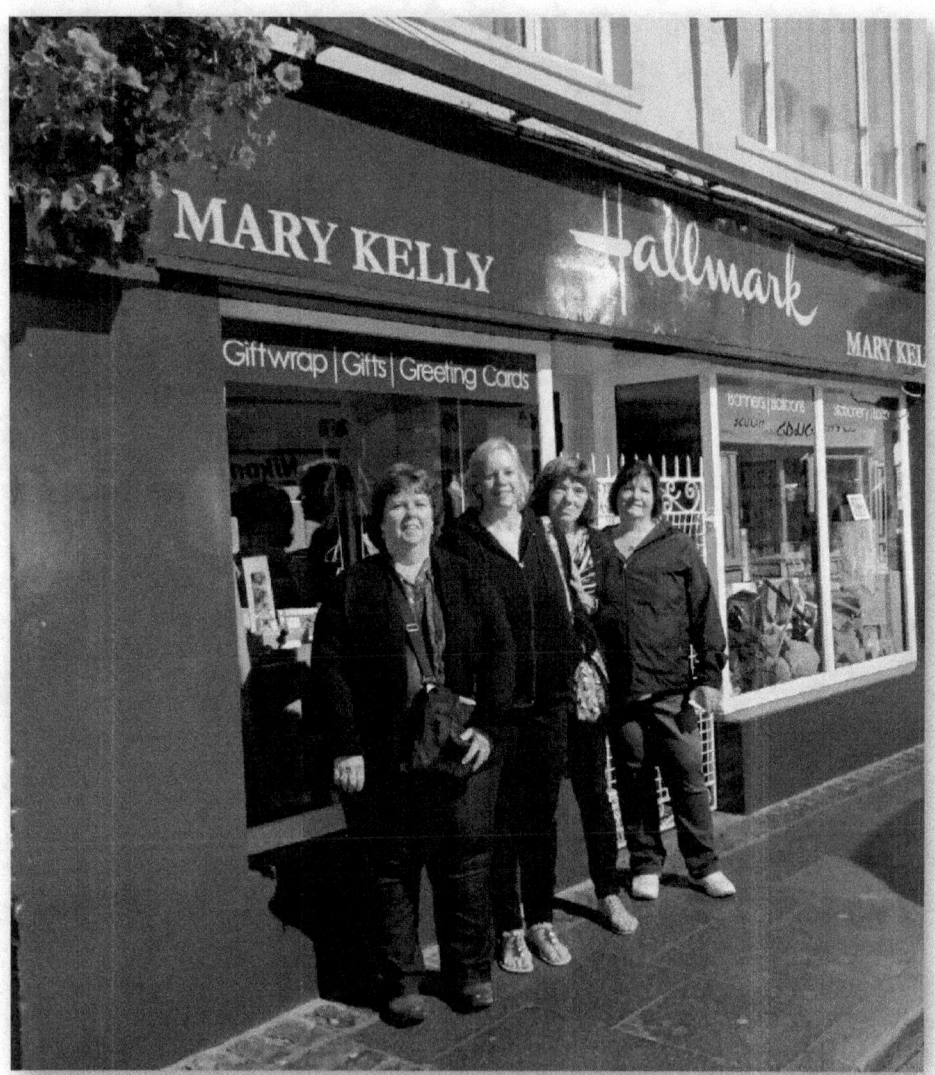

Mary Kelly Adams passed in 2015 but she is still with us. We saw this store in Ennis, Ireland on the last night of our trip there in August 2017. Coincidence? I don't think so. Madam loved Hallmark stores and we had been talking about her all week. I truly believe this was a sign from her.

Madam, you will always be with us!

From left, Terry S., Me, Terri B, and Mary C.